# Regaining
## Your Self

# Also by Ira M. Sacker, M.D.

*Dying to Be Thin: Understanding and
Defeating Anorexia Nervosa and Bulimia—
A Practical, Lifesaving Guide*
(with Marc A. Zimmer, Ph.D.)

# Regaining
## Your Self

UNDERSTANDING AND CONQUERING

THE EATING DISORDER IDENTITY

## IRA M. SACKER, M.D.

Coauthor of *Dying to Be Thin*

with Sheila Buff

Health Communications, Inc.
Deerfield Beach, Florida

*www.hcibooks.com*

The information in this book is not intended to be a substitute for the medical advice of a physician. Readers should consult with their doctors in all matters relating to health and for treatment of their medical problems. Although every effort has been made to ensure that information is presented accurately in this book, the ultimate responsibility for proper medical treatment rests with the prescribing physician, in consultation and partnership with the reader. Neither the publisher nor the authors assume any responsibility for errors or for any possible consequences arising from the use of information contained herein.

**Library of Congress Cataloging-in-Publication Data is available through the Library of Congress.**

Copyright © 2007, 2010 Ira M. Sacker, M.D.
ISBN-13: 978-07573-1501-5
ISBN-10: 0-7573-1501-1

Hardcover edition published by Hyperion, 2007. ISBN-13: 978-1-4013-0305-1; ISBN-10: 1-4013-0305-6

Publisher: Health Communications, Inc.
  3201 S.W. 15th Street
  Deerfield Beach, FL 33442–8190

*Cover design by Lawna Patterson Oldfield*
*Inside book design by Jennifer Daddio*
*Workbook formatted by Dawn Von Strolley Grove*

Marianne Sacker is my wife, my best friend, my partner in life, my companion, and my advocate. My guiding spirit and my true soul mate, Marianne has protected me in times of weakness, believed in me during times of doubt, inspired me during my creative moments, and with her constant, loving reassurance continues to teach me the values of humility and giving to others. Our relationship and marriage, built on forty-plus years, have taught me honesty, sincerity, and loyalty. Marianne's compassion, love, and selflessness during all these years have never gone unnoticed. It's her joy for life that has kept my spirit young and is the centerpiece of her unique sense of self.

Without Marianne my life would not be complete; she balances my days and my nights.

*To love someone deeply*
*gives you strength.*
*Being loved by someone*
*deeply gives you courage.*

—LAO TZU

A trusted colleague and friend, Laura D. McDonald, M.S., has been a major contributor to this work. Her constant pursuit of clarity and excellence gave this book heart and soul. Her contributions to the writing, editing, and development of theory deserve special recognition. Through our conversations together we have both brought life to this book. This dedication is a small token to the total contribution that Laura has made, not just throughout this book, but in the field of eating disorders. And for that I would like to express my gratitude.

*The bond that links*
*your true family is not one of blood,*
*but of respect and joy in each other's life.*
*Rarely do members of one family*
*grow up under the same roof.*

— RICHARD BACH

# CONTENTS

# AUTHOR'S NOTE

*Throughout the writing* of this book I have tried to faithfully represent the struggle of individuals with eating disorders as I have witnessed them through my more than thirty-five years of working in the field. There are, however, difficulties, as accurate portrayals of these disorders may sometimes prove to be triggers to the very people who are struggling against them. That is why, whenever possible, I have avoided the use of specific numbers such as pounds, calories, amount of weight loss or weight gain, and so on. For the same reason, I have not provided information or specifics as to certain at-risk behaviors and activities. Whatever insight one reader may experience in being privy to such details would be nothing compared to the anxiety another may feel, to say nothing of the risk. As always, it is my job to protect the individual suffering from, or at risk of, an eating disorder.

The stories contained within these pages are true. Names have been changed to protect the privacy of the individuals concerned. While some case studies represent composite characters, their stories are never exaggerated or overstated.

Because I strongly believe that identity is the core issue of the eating disorder, I have tried not to use labels like "anorexic" and "bulimic," as to do so would only reinforce the eating disorder identity, and have used instead phrases such as "the individual who struggles with . . ." or "the person with. . . ."

This book is the result of many years of work. I sincerely hope that it helps you, and invite you to visit my website for further information: www.sackermd.com.

# ACKNOWLEDGMENTS

*I would first* like to thank the two individuals who gave me life, my parents. My father, Harvey, who always made me feel safe, encouraged me throughout medical school and taught me my greatest passion—fishing.

My mother, Lottie, who showed me immeasurable strength and how to survive and never lose hope through all the obstacles of life. She taught me more than anything to always believe in myself.

My wife, Marianne, completes my life with her love, companionship, and spirit. She has given me many gifts in life, but watching her be a wife, mother, and grandmother is the biggest gift of all. Her ability to be an independent individual strengthens everyone around her.

Remembering my little sister Karen. She was my fishing buddy, and no matter who began fishing first, she always caught the first fish. In many respects I was a guardian to this individual throughout her years in this world.

My son, Scott, is an independent spirit. He has been one of my best teachers. He has taught me the meaning of change and how to be an effective parent and teacher by example.

My daughter, Tara, is always enthusiastic and passionate about life.

She has taught me that the value of love we have shared with our children she now shares with her own children.

Tara and her husband, Owen, have given me the gift of grandparenthood. My grandchildren, Michael and Dylan, call me "Popi." My greatest joy is being with my grandchildren, playing with them, spoiling them, and ultimately giving them back to their parents.

I want to recognize my family and friends throughout the years who have taught me many lessons through laughter and tears.

I want to acknowledge two of my mentors: Dr. Saul Krugman and Dr. Edward Liang.

I would like to thank Laura D. McDonald, M.S., for her thoughts, concepts, organized ideas, therapeutic modalities/charts, creative narratives, and precision for words. I also thank her for her willingness to share personal perspectives that are enmeshed throughout this book; without her and her dedication, this book would never have been written.

Finally, I want to acknowledge all the individuals who struggle every day with an eating disorder and the ones who have recovered their identities from an eating disorder. I want to honor the families and friends who are devoted in the fight against the epidemic.

I would like to continue my support to the organizations and individuals who are fighting to make the difference in ending eating disorders.

Finally, I would like to express my gratitude to all the professionals who work in this field and make an impact in the lives they touch.

*Just when the caterpillar*
*thought the world was over,*
*it became a butterfly.*

—ANONYMOUS

# Discovering the Self

*My first patient* with anorexia was sixteen years old and on the brink of death from malnutrition. I had no idea what to do.

Until a few days before, I had been a young resident in pediatrics at New York University Medical Center and Bellevue Hospital Center. On that day in 1970, I was a brand-new fellow in adolescent medicine at Los Angeles Children's Hospital. I had arrived at the hospital first thing that morning, bleary eyed and jet-lagged, expecting to spend the day meeting the big shots who had started this pioneering program. Instead, when I introduced myself to the head nurse, she said, "Your patient is waiting for you on the adolescent floor."

"Excuse me?" I said. "Isn't there some sort of orientation I need to have first?"

"We'll get to the orientation later," she replied. "They want you up there now."

I was a little surprised and not feeling particularly confident, but I was eager to make a good impression and begin work in my new position. I was also so new to the hospital that I had to ask how to get to the adolescent floor. From inside the elevator as it approached the ninth floor, I could hear enraged screaming. As I arrived in the reception area, I saw where all the noise was coming from: A teenaged girl was in a hair-pulling tug-of-war with her mother, all the while cursing her at the top of her lungs. The mother seized the girl's handbag and turned it upside down. Dozens of tiny white pills spilled out all over the floor.

I knew right away this was my patient. I was still a young doctor back then, but I had been in medicine long enough to realize that the hospital staff had dealt with this girl before. They knew I was coming and were taking advantage of the new guy by passing a difficult patient off to me.

The nurse behind the reception desk took one look at me and pointed at the battle going on before us. "You must be Dr. Sacker," she said. "That's Julia. You can use exam room A."

I somehow managed to get Julia and her mother into the exam room without getting punched in the process. When I was able to take a closer look at Julia, I was shocked. This blue-eyed, blond girl was about five foot four and terribly underweight. She looked as if every bone in her body could break at any moment. She was so thin I couldn't understand how she could even stand up, much less put up such a fight. In fact, I couldn't really understand why she wasn't dead.

Putting on my best professional manner, I introduced myself: "Hi, I'm Dr. Sacker, the new fellow in adolescent medicine."

Her response was short and to the point: "I don't want to talk to you." Then she resumed screaming at her mother.

Still using my best professional manner to cover the mounting panic I was feeling, I tried to get her to calm down. I looked over to her mother and realized immediately that there wasn't going to be any help there. Julia's mother was in shock and clearly needed someone else to handle this. All I could get out of her was that her daughter had been diagnosed with anorexia nervosa—a disease I had vaguely heard of but never seen, much less treated.

I tried again and still couldn't get through to Julia. I couldn't even begin to take a history. Finally, I sent her mother out of the room, and Julia calmed down enough for me to get some much-needed information. She told me those tiny white pills were to suppress her hunger. I told her she needed to be hospitalized, now.

She looked at me, laughed, and refused—totally, absolutely, adamantly.

I was at a loss. If this girl didn't get medical attention at once, she was going to die. I called my supervising physician (whom I had yet to meet face-to-face). Trying to sound competent and unflustered, I told him my patient was out of control, needed immediate treatment, and was refusing voluntary admission. What was I supposed to do now?

He told me that if she obviously needed treatment but was refusing admission, she had to be sent to the county hospital's general psychiatric unit. The procedure, he said, was to call a county ambulance. The attendants would come and put her in restraints; then they would drive off with her, and with any luck I'd never see her again.

Great, I thought. It's not even nine in the morning of my first day and I'm having my first patient put into restraints and sent off in an ambulance. I followed procedure. Julia was taken away. Her mother left. Okay, not my problem anymore—next patient, please.

I spent the rest of the day seeing adolescents in the outpatient clinic, and by the end of the day I felt like a real doctor again. I was also completely wiped out from the combination of stress and jet lag. I went home to my new apartment and collapsed into bed.

At three in the morning, the phone rang. It was a state police officer. He told me that he had a missing person named Julia in custody. She had managed to escape from the county psych unit and make her way home to her mother's house. Her mother, however, had refused to let her in, and Julia had then proceeded to break every window in the house. That was amazing enough, but what the officer said next just astonished me: "She says you're her doctor. What do you want to do?"

Good question, I thought. "Put her on the phone."

"I'll come to the hospital," Julia said. I didn't have to say anything. She had clearly figured out for herself that between the county psychiatric unit and me, I was the better choice.

The next morning, Julia was waiting for me. She was calm, controlled, and ready to be admitted. At this point, understandably, it was her mother who was the wreck. We once again went into an exam room, and now Julia was willing to give me her medical history. She had been restricting her food intake and using appetite suppressants for more than eighteen months. She had lost forty pounds.

I told her that while I could treat her medically and save her from dying of self-starvation, she also needed psychiatric care. I very frankly told her that I didn't know anything about anorexia. As it turned out, the psychiatrist who was called in to evaluate her didn't know anything about anorexia either. In 1970, very few did.

Julia's psychiatrist gave her large doses of heavy-duty tranquilizers while I worked out a nutrition plan that would gradually help her regain weight without causing additional medical problems. At first we had to give her a liquid formula using a nasogastric tube—an unpleasant procedure for everyone.

During the first week Julia was on the adolescent floor, I was very worried about her. I was afraid she would die of severe malnutrition despite our efforts. It was clear from the start that her sole goal and interest in life was to lose as much weight as she possibly could. Other than that, all I could tell about her was that she was an angry young woman.

She refused to talk to the psychiatrist, saying instead that she wanted to talk to me. But I protested, saying, "I don't know anything about anorexia. I don't think I can help you." And yet, at the same time, I felt drawn to Julia—something about her behavior reminded me of myself. My own adolescence hadn't been easy, and deep down I thought I understood, at least a little, how she felt. Like me at that age, she had not a clue as to her own identity.

Finally I did something I knew I wasn't supposed to do, something that went against all my years of medical training. I was taught to ask the questions and wait for the responses from the patient, and to never, ever reveal anything about myself. Julia wasn't buying it. She simply wouldn't talk to me that way—she would sit there and refuse to say a word. After a week of this I was so frustrated that I just began chatting to her, telling her that I was originally from California, that I was in L.A. to learn about adolescent medicine, and that I knew next to nothing about eating disorders. Before I knew it, we had formed some sort of bond and she started opening up to me.

After two months on the adolescent floor, Julia had finally gained enough weight to be discharged. Her parents thought that because she had gained weight, she was well. So did I.

Julia continued to see me on an outpatient basis three times a week for medical exams and weight checks. She came faithfully but immediately started to lose weight. I warned her that if she lost three more pounds she would have to go back into the hospital. That got through to her, I thought, and her weight immediately stabilized. There was just one problem: as the next three weeks went by, the scale stayed the same, yet I could see that she was getting thinner and thinner.

I was slow on the uptake, but I finally caught on to the ways she was fooling the scale. When I was able to get her real weight, she had managed to lose six pounds. That meant being readmitted to the adolescent floor for another round of inpatient treatment. This time I was less worried about losing her, and she was more open with me. I began to like her as a person: a lonely person who had been emotionally abused by an angry mother and had almost no relationship at all with her father. I discovered that hiding beneath the anorexia was a very bright young woman and an outstanding student. Despite her excellent grades, she never really felt she was good enough—the only way she could cope with the pressures of life and feel under control was to stop eating.

At the time I didn't really know what I did to help Julia, but she regained the weight quickly and was discharged in three weeks. As before, I continued to see her three times a week in the outpatient clinic. She still met with the nutritionist and was weighed, but when we talked, we no longer discussed her weight and food. Instead, we chatted about her—who she was, what her interests were. In these relaxed sessions, we enjoyed each other's company. Her smarts came out, her fears were no longer there, she was finally able to talk about the underlying issue of her feelings of inadequacy. We talked about everything *but* her weight. She told me she wanted to be an actress but her mother didn't want her to. I told her that I had wanted to be an actor but my father wouldn't allow it. Now we really had something in common.

Julia wanted to return to school so she could graduate and go on to college. Her high school, however, had failed her for missing so many days.

Doctors aren't usually supposed to get involved with this sort of thing, but I called the school and managed to get them to readmit her and let her transition in by attending just a few hours each day. By the time my fellowship was over and I had to return to New York, Julia had made up her schoolwork and had been accepted to college—with a scholarship.

During my six months in Los Angeles, I ended up treating several other patients with eating disorders as well. The county psychiatric hospital heard about Julia and started sending me other teenaged patients with eating disorders. At first I thought that was because I had been so successful with Julia, but I quickly realized it was because they just wanted these difficult, dangerously ill patients out of their hospital.

I saw these teens as purely medical cases. Mostly I worried about making sure they didn't die—I didn't pay a lot of attention to their emotional problems. It didn't strike me until near the end of my fellowship that there were a lot of similarities between who my patients were and who I was, that I had all the dynamics of a patient with an eating disorder. I was an overachiever, I was perfectionistic, I had my own level of obsessive-compulsive traits. When I was studying for exams, for instance, I didn't know when to stop. No matter how many good grades I got, the euphoria lasted for only a few seconds. Then my mind would take me to the next level of obsessive studying. My patients were the same way—their expectations of themselves were completely overwhelming. Looking at these patients was like looking in a mirror.

If you had told me, back in those early days, that I would be spending all my time treating patients with eating disorders, I would have said, no way, no how. I couldn't even find any information about anorexia so I could learn more—it just didn't exist then. My treatment method for my patients was improvised out of anxiety, not knowledge. Fortunately, none of them died and none of them relapsed. I thought I had found an effective approach, but what I really had were young patients, early diagnosis, and not much cultural pressure to be thin. There was nothing positive in society to reinforce the eating disorder behavior. But mostly, I got lucky. I was able to be a talker, a listener, and a healer all at the same time—exactly why I had gone into medicine.

When I returned to New York, I still thought eating disorder patients were rare, something that in ordinary practice I would encounter only occasionally. I was wrong—the epidemic of eating disorders was just beginning to escalate.

As part of my medical education arrangements, I had to do three years of military service. I was sent to Frankfurt, Germany, to run a pediatric/adolescent medicine program for military families at the large army base there. While I was there, I developed a comprehensive healthcare program called the Youth Health Center. The three years I spent working with these adolescents really opened my eyes. The pressures they faced—drugs, alcohol, sex, family breakups, fears for parents sent into danger—were way beyond anything I had faced growing up. What I discovered from the Youth Health Center was the importance of being open-minded and nonjudgmental. I also learned how a transitional setting within the community could create a place where patients could gradually move from a hospital setting back to an independent life.

I took the lessons from Frankfurt back to New York with me. It was 1975 and I was now the chief of adolescent medicine at Brookdale University Hospital and Medical Center—a primary affiliate of the New York University Medical Center at the time. We were pioneering the whole concept of adolescent medicine.

I began to get referrals for young patients with eating disorders, and soon I was admitting new eating disorder patients. By 1980 the numbers had increased so dramatically that we had to expand the inpatient adolescent division to incorporate the treatment of acute eating disorders.

Suddenly eating disorders were a major topic in adolescent medicine. Papers started appearing in professional journals. Hilde Bruch's groundbreaking book *The Golden Cage* appeared in 1978, and then the floodgates of popular books, magazine articles, TV shows, movies, and more opened. Anorexia and bulimia were hot topics. The problem, from my point of view, was that everything I was reading in the professional literature, everything I was hearing at medical conferences, seemed to differ from what I was observing with my own patients. The early experts were saying eating disorders were rooted in the external struggle for control between parent and child. They were saying girls became anorexic as a way to avoid their own sexuality. They were saying eating disorders were rooted in childhood trauma.

If the causes of eating disorders were confusing, the treatment recommendations were even more complicated. We all had a pretty good idea of how to deal with the medical issues of severely malnourished patients, but beyond that, the approaches were all over the place, with advocates for each claiming they had the right answer.

I kept reading all the material and going to all the conferences, and I kept trying to apply the latest analytic approaches to my patients, but they seldom worked. Following the most authoritative thinking of the time, we started to use a behavioral program. Eating disorder patients were admitted to the hospital and put in a restrictive environment. The more they cooperated and gained weight, the more specific privileges were returned to them. The approach seemed to work well—patients quickly caught on to the system, complied with the routine, and gained enough weight to be discharged. At first, everyone—doctors, nurses, parents, patients—was extremely hopeful. But then we started to have repeat customers. Adolescents who had been discharged at reasonable weights were being readmitted, sometimes just a few months later, dangerously underweight again. It soon became clear to me that they had gained weight just to comply with the program. Once they were out of the hospital and back into their community, the symptoms quickly returned. Not only was the behavioral approach not working, I felt it was actually making things worse.

I kept falling back to the approach that seemed so natural to me: just talking and listening to these patients. They opened up to me and began to share the things that really interested them—the things that told them who they really were. Somehow, this method helped them begin to let go of their eating disorders. I came to realize that for many of my patients, the eating disorder filled a huge identity void in their lives. By helping them discover something else—some passionate interest rooted in their own personalities and talents—to fill that void, we ultimately replaced the power of the eating disorder.

I found that my patients responded best when I went in with an open mind, willing to do anything to help them. I tried to develop an individual relationship with each patient, to understand their distinct personality and to tailor the treatment to fit their individual needs. And the more I treated my patients as individuals, the more they became individuals.

What seems to work best for my patients is an approach to therapy that combines three aspects: personal, interactive, and rational. In our sessions I'm not distant from my patients and I don't see them as just cases—they're real people, and I've found that they respond best when I reveal aspects of my personality to them. Our sessions are interactive. The rational aspect of therapy is crucial. Eating disorder patients generally can't see themselves clearly—they need a therapist's help to see the reality of their condition and to grasp the ways out of it.

I call this approach personal interactive rational therapy, or PIRT for short. PIRT is based on the insights I've gained from years of experience in treating eating disorders. PIRT provides a framework for successful treatment. I know from my own patients and those of my colleagues that patients get better when they develop a strong personal relationship with the therapist, based on mutual openness, trust, and respect.

*By the 1980s,* as the eating disorder epidemic grew and the media became more interested, I felt I had something to add to the existing literature on eating disorders. In 1987 I coauthored a book about anorexia and bulimia, *Dying to Be Thin,* that received a great deal of national recognition. And by the 1990s, when the eating disorder epidemic had become even worse, I started to get calls from reporters and talk show producers for interviews about this expanding epidemic. Soon I was on television on a regular basis and getting constant calls from reporters—a demand that continues to this day.

In my media appearances I try not to exploit individuals with eating disorders but rather to educate our society about the importance of prevention, awareness, and treatment. I have been a guest expert on shows such as *The Oprah Winfrey Show, Good Morning America,* the *Today* show, *CNN News, 48 Hours, 60 Minutes,* and more. In every interview, on every TV show, in every publication, I talk about the role of identity and a strong sense of self in preventing eating disorders. I talk about how a passion in life can replace the eating disorder and fill the inner void it once occupied. And I talk about how individuals with eating disorders, even long-standing ones, can be helped.

In 2005, after thirty years at Brookdale University Hospital and Medical Center, the time had come to step down. Today I'm a visiting clinical professor at New York University Medical Center and Bellevue Hospital Center. I continue my mission of helping to end eating disorders through my well-established private practice in Manhattan and Long Island, New York. Through the stories and insights my patients have given me over the years, I hope to share my philosophy and treatment approach as an eating disorder specialist.

# ONE

# Identifying the Disorder

*In my thirty-five*-plus years of practice, only one patient has ever told me she wanted to have an eating disorder. Only one person has walked through my door and said, "I made a conscious decision to become anorexic." Every other patient I've ever treated found herself unintentionally ensnared by an eating disorder, the result of any number of influences, decisions, and circumstances.

The desire for weight loss is the most common starting point for an eating disorder. It can begin innocently enough, with the desire to lose weight and look better. But for some people the physical changes that weight loss brings about are so seductive, the praise they receive from others is so gratifying, that they feel compelled to further diet. Changes in brain chemistry brought about by weight loss can also reinforce these limits, and, as if something is set in motion, an eating disorder is soon in place. Other factors may also come into play. Having an illness that leads to appetite loss and weight loss may start an eating disorder. A significant change in circumstances, such as a divorce, a death in the family, or a move, can make an individual vulnerable. Positive events such as a wedding or a new job may also be responsible. Sometimes, people will restrict (or, in the opposite direction, binge) in an attempt to combat anxiety, and possibly depression. And sometimes, even an offhand remark like "You've put on a few pounds" can be enough to get someone started down the road to an eating disorder. Whatever the trigger, it's important to know that eating disorders do not come about by choice.

# How Does It Start?

Ironically, the eating disorder, which can represent a profound threat to a person's health, can often be traced back to a desire at first to become healthier, a desire that finds expression in a weight-loss diet and sometimes exercise. Most people who decide to go on a diet end up following a script that has a predictable ending. The dieter will adhere to the advice given in just about every diet book—restrict food intake and exercise more—and that generally works for about the first month or so. The first couple of weeks are very gratifying because most people will lose several pounds quickly. The next couple of weeks are harder—the weight comes off more slowly, and the hunger pains and sense of deprivation grow. By the end of the month, the dieter has lost perhaps ten pounds, but weight loss has stalled. At that point the denials and rationalizations begin: "One cookie won't make a difference." "I've been so good I deserve this treat." "I'll take a break today and be good tomorrow." The diet and exercise stop. The lost weight gradually returns.

---

*For some people, going on a weight-loss diet seems to trigger something in them. They find a deep satisfaction in restriction and a deep gratification in weight loss. For these people, the sense of accomplishment that comes with weight loss, along with the praise and admiration they receive as a result, gives them a new identity, the identity of someone who's really good at being disciplined and losing weight.*

---

For others, however, the physical changes in the body offer concrete evidence that efforts are paying off. This is motivating, as is the realization that the cause and effect of diet and weight loss are straightforward in a way that little else is. But as she restricts her diet more and more, as she loses more and more weight, any tendencies the person might have

# A Spectrum Disorder

Eating disorders range across a spectrum. At one end are people with extreme anorexia who severely restrict their food intake; at the other are binge eaters and compulsive overeaters who can't control their desire to eat large quantities of food. Also included in that spectrum are people with bulimia, who may binge on food and then purge by vomiting, overexercising, or using laxatives or diuretics. The intensity of a disorder can change over time for each individual, and often the distinctions between one category and another are blurred. Eating disorders are generally associated with extreme weight loss and emaciation from anorexia, but in reality anorexia is just one aspect of the broader eating disorder spectrum. In fact, someone who's overweight could become anorexic or might turn to bulimic behavior and still appear overweight.

What all patients with eating disorders have in common is an inability to see themselves as they are. While these people can generally look at others and see that they're a normal weight, or too thin or too heavy, when they look at themselves they see only a distorted image. One end of the spectrum is significantly underweight, while the other end of the spectrum is significantly overweight. Throughout the entire spectrum the mirror consistently gives a distorted reflection to someone with any eating disorder.

toward obsessive-compulsive disorder and perfectionism, two common characteristics of individuals with eating disorders, have an opportunity to really blossom. And as she loses more and more weight, she discovers something else. Weight loss feels good because it helps to calm the high level of anxiety that is another common characteristic of individuals with eating disorders. Being in a state of semistarvation causes changes in the metabolism and brain chemistry that reinforce the restricting behavior by creating a natural high. Further reinforcement comes from family and friends, especially peers. They're all saying, "Wow, you look great" and "I really admire all your hard work." Now the person is not only feeling the high but also getting all this reinforcement. It appears to be a win-win situation, but the end result is a serious eating disorder.

# Defining the Disorder

By the time a patient ends up in my office, the eating disorder has generally been in place for months, if not years. It can take that long for a parent, spouse, or friend to realize that an eating disorder has taken root. It can take weeks or even months longer to convince the patient that treatment is needed, and then it can take weeks, months, or even years to find the right sort of treatment. In the meantime, of course, the eating disorder only grows stronger, as does the damage it causes.

The sooner an eating disorder is recognized, the easier it is to treat the problem. I know from experience, however, that individuals with eating disorders become very adept at hiding them. Even specialists can fail to see an eating disorder when it first presents itself. Definitions are a big

---

*Eating disorders don't start overnight, although they can progress quickly once they take hold. In most cases, the illness comes on slowly and quietly, unnoticed both by the patient and the community.*

---

part of the problem in detecting these disorders early on. At what point does being on a diet or eating too much become classified as a disorder? At what point does the desire for exercise cross over into an obsession? At what point does the act of taking refuge in "comfort food" turn into a binge eating disorder? It's a fine line, and often the patient is well across it before anyone notices.

## Anorexia Nervosa

I recently started seeing a patient named Tessa. She's thirty-five and has a long treatment history. Before coming to see me, she had been treated by no less than eight different physicians and therapists specializing in eating disorders. According to Tessa, not one had the same eating disorder diagnosis for her and none were very effective in treating her. She was willing to give treatment one last try, which was why she was in my office.

At our first session, Tessa shared some of her early history. She was diagnosed with anorexia nervosa when she was fourteen, when she restricted her diet so much that she lost a significant amount of weight and stopped having her period. At that point, Tessa had all the major behavior patterns of the disease known as anorexia nervosa, as defined by the latest *Diagnostic and Statistical Manual of Mental Disorders* (DSM) published by the American Psychiatric Association. These are the standard guidelines used by therapists, physicians, psychiatrists, psychologists, treatment programs, and others to define eating disorders. They're not perfect, but they're widely accepted as a workable way to ensure that everyone is defining the various eating disorders in more or less the same way.

In high school, Tessa showed all the classic signs of anorexia. She restricted her food intake so much that she had severe weight loss that was greater than 15 percent of the normal body weight for someone of her age and height. (Older definitions of anorexia nervosa said the weight loss had to be 25 percent or more—we're making some progress in diagnosing the disorder sooner.)

*The DSM provides the standard guidelines used by therapists, physicians, psychiatrists, psychologists, treatment programs, and others to define eating disorders. They're not perfect, but they're widely accepted as a workable way to ensure that everyone is defining the various eating disorders in more or less the same way.*

At fourteen, Tessa had starved herself down to a severely anorexic weight. Painfully thin, she also had many of the physical problems caused by severe weight loss: fatigue, hair loss, brittle nails, black circles under her eyes, low blood pressure, a slowed heart rate, easy bruising, thinning bones (osteopenia), and low body temperature (hypothermia). As well, she had many of the emotional and physical complications: severe mood swings, depression, generalized aches and pains, agitation and anxiety, and sleep disturbances. Tessa also had another very serious psychological problem: frequent thoughts of suicide. Although she never acted on them, her suicidal thoughts were extremely upsetting and unnerving.

Like everyone with anorexia, Tessa absolutely refused to gain weight. No amount of discussion, persuasion, bribing, yelling, or threatening could make her eat more. Tessa's family, her family doctor, and her therapist tried everything but couldn't get through to her. She also had a seriously distorted body image. (People with anorexia usually see themselves as fat even when they are clearly very underweight. In addition, they usually deny how serious their low weight is.) Tessa was convinced she was fat even when her weight did not reflect that image.

Tessa also had another important sign that applies to females with anorexia nervosa: She stopped having menstrual periods. A female is diagnosed anorexic if she's missed three consecutive periods because her body weight is too low. Tessa went almost two years without having a period.

*The formal definition of anorexia nervosa doesn't give any age guidelines. Anorexia generally starts between the ages of about eleven and fourteen, but I've seen anorexic patients in their forties and fifties. I've even seen them as young as five. Anorexia is often thought of as a disease of teenaged girls, but today more and more young men and older women are being diagnosed with it as well as other eating disorders. The face of anorexia—and of all eating disorders—has changed in recent years to include a broader range of ages, more men, and more minority group members.*

Within the anorexia nervosa diagnosis, there are two types: restricting types and binge-eating/purging types. Restricting types will rigidly limit their intake to small and smaller amounts of food. Binge-eating/purging types will usually restrict during the day, followed by eating large amounts of food in binges in the evening, then purging by vomiting or misusing laxatives and diuretics. (The binge-eating/purging type of anorexia differs from bulimia in that the binge and purge are not planned and the individual can still restrict food intake.) Tessa was classified as the restricting type of anorexic.

Tessa stayed anorexic until she was a senior in high school, when she finally began to eat more and gain weight. This is not an uncommon pattern. Young women with anorexia do sometimes seem to just get over it, but that's often an illusion. In many cases, what has really happened is that the eating disorder has simply taken another form. Tessa ate more and gained weight, but because she was afraid her weight gain would get out of control, she started running. That quickly grew into an obsession, and she advanced rapidly from short distances to marathons. Her weight dropped back to her anorexic levels as her running became more obsessive and ritualistic.

## Bulimia: Binge and Purge

When she was forced to restrict her physical activity, Tessa's solution was bulimia: She binged on certain very specific foods and then purged by making herself vomit. This was a very different behavior pattern from her earlier anorexia.

Obsessive exercise as a way to burn off additional calories isn't part of the formal definitions of eating disorders in the DSM, but in my experience about half of all my patients will engage in excessive exercise, called exercise bulimia. Tessa certainly fit into that part of bulimic behavior. Eventually the excessive exercise, combined with poor nutrition, caused a stress fracture in her ankle and Tessa had to stop running. The sudden lack of physical activity sent her into a severe depression and made her obsess again about weight gain.

The difference between someone with anorexia and someone with bulimia is that individuals with bulimia are usually normal weight or even overweight—they're generally not significantly underweight. When I started treating Tessa, she was close to normal weight, even though she was bingeing and purging several times a week. Repeated binge eating is very typical of someone with bulimia. During her binges, Tessa would eat several large bags of chips—far more than is normal. Even while she was eating them, she knew her eating was out of control, but she couldn't stop. So, to control her weight between binges, Tessa would make herself throw up. She also misused laxatives and diuretics and would sometimes starve herself in between binges. Once her ankle healed and she was able

---

*Obsessive exercise as a way to burn off additional calories isn't part of the formal definitions of eating disorders in the DSM, but in my experience about half of all my patients will engage in excessive exercise, called exercise bulimia.*

---

to exercise again, Tessa went back to obsessive exercise, on a treadmill. Needless to say, she remained excessively concerned with her weight and body image.

Bulimia has two types: purging and nonpurging. Tessa was the purging type, which is much more common. People with nonpurging bulimia generally do vomit on occasion, but most attempt to control their weight between binges by excessive exercise.

Bulimia is a disease that tends to start at a somewhat later age than anorexia. For most of my patients with bulimia, the behavior began between the ages of fourteen and eighteen. It may occur in pockets—among the members of a college sorority, for instance—but you certainly don't have to be a college student to have it. Older people who, like Tessa, have an earlier history of anorexia can become bulimic. Although most patients feel, at least at first, that bulimia is a way to "have their cake and eat it, too," they don't usually realize that bulimia also carries a serious risk of severe complications and even sudden death.

Bulimia often causes weight loss when the behavior first starts—that's why many patients become so attached to it. As the behavior continues, however, the body's own physiology kicks in and tries to stop the weight loss. The body's overall metabolism slows down as a way to preserve calories. The digestion process in the mouth kicks into overdrive and increases the digestion even before the food is swallowed. The swollen salivary glands this causes are what give someone with bulimia chipmunk cheeks. The acid from frequent vomiting causes stomach problems and severe damage to the teeth; loss of electrolytes, which includes potassium, can lead to cardiac arrest or sudden death.

---

*The difference between someone with anorexia and someone with bulimia is that individuals with bulimia are usually normal weight or even overweight—they're generally not significantly underweight.*

---

## Eating Disorder Not Otherwise Specified

When Tessa began seeing me, she was almost a textbook example of purging-type bulimia. When she described herself in high school, it was almost like reading the textbook definition of anorexia nervosa. But over the years, her eating disorder behavior had varied, sometimes tending more toward anorexia, sometimes more toward bulimia, and occasionally getting somewhat better. That had led some of her therapists during this time to give her my least favorite diagnosis: Eating Disorder Not Otherwise Specified, or ED NOS.

This is a catchall diagnosis that has often confused doctors as well as therapists. They know the patient has some sort of problem related to food and eating, and they know they have to put some sort of diagnosis into the chart. This is what happened to Tessa several times; it's why she had seen so many different doctors and therapists over the years and still didn't recover.

Officially, a diagnosis of ED NOS means the patient has problems related to appetite, eating, body image, and body weight, but that those problems don't meet the criteria for anorexia and bulimia as I've just described them. It could be that the patient really has some other sort of mental illness, such as depression or possibly even schizophrenia. It's also possible she has a medical problem, such as irritable bowel syndrome or Crohn's disease, that leads to weight loss, vomiting, diarrhea, and other symptoms that could be similar to those of an eating disorder. A competent physician would rule those out before deciding on the NOS label. In my experience, however, most patients who are labeled as NOS really are already anorexic or bulimic—it's just that they haven't yet developed the full range of symptoms. Let's say a patient has many of the other symptoms of anorexia, such

---

*You don't have to be underweight to have an eating disorder.*

---

as restricting her diet and having a distorted body image, but she's still getting her period. That's usually just because her weight loss isn't so extreme yet that her body shuts down her hormone production. In my book she's anorexic, and the sooner we start treatment, the better.

On the other hand, some patients clearly have an eating disorder that's not exactly anorexia or bulimia. A good example of having an eating disorder NOS would be patients we call "spitters." These patients show a lot of bulimic behavior in terms of eating small or large amounts of food at a time, but they don't actually swallow the food; instead they chew it up and spit it out. That means they don't later try to get rid of the food by vomiting, purging, or exercise. They're not really bulimic, but they still have an eating disorder that needs immediate treatment.

My biggest objection to the "not otherwise specified" category is that all too often, patients and family members think that it means the patient doesn't really have an eating disorder at all. When that happens, they tend to think that somehow the problem has been defined away and that treatment isn't needed. This is when patients can fall between the cracks, not get the help they need, and even end up dead from the consequences of the eating disorder, or from suicide.

Whenever the diagnosis is ED NOS, it's extremely important to convince everyone that there still is a significant problem that needs to be addressed. I've had a number of patients who didn't want to be classified as "not otherwise specified" but rather be classified as having an eating disorder. One patient, Autumn, really stands out in that area. At forty-two, she's extremely thin and appears emaciated, but she's medically stable. Her blood work is acceptable: no anemia, no electrolyte imbalances, for example. Her bone density is, just barely, normal for someone her age. The clincher, from Autumn's perspective, is that although she has been this thin for years, she maintains regular periods. Whenever I use the word "anorexia" with her, Autumn quotes the DSM definition to me and says, "I'm not anorexic because I still get my period. Plus my doctor says I'm fine." Technically speaking, she's right. The formal diagnosis has to be ED NOS. But defining the problem as something other than anorexia doesn't actually make it go away.

## Overeating Disorders

Two major eating disorders involve overeating. Binge eating disorder (BED) is characterized by periods of uncontrolled eating, where large quantities of food (often a specific "favorite" food) are consumed in a short time. Unlike bulimia, however, BED involves only bingeing; it's not followed by purging or any other attempt to "get rid" of the food. Individuals with BED often feel out of control during the binge. They know that they're harming themselves, and they often eat to the point of being uncomfortably full, but they also can't stop. They usually eat alone, and often in secret. Not surprisingly, the binge episode is usually followed by intense feelings of guilt, shame, and depression. Most individuals with binge eating disorder are overweight and struggle to lose weight.

Compulsive overeating is a somewhat different eating disorder. These individuals are generally overweight and feel addicted to food, us-

## A Dangerous Disease

Eating disorders have the highest mortality rate of any mental illness. About 20 percent of all patients with anorexia nervosa will die either as a direct result of the disorder or by suicide. In anorexia, death comes from self-starvation; in bulimia, death can come suddenly from a ruptured esophagus or the loss of potassium caused by excessive vomiting, resulting in sudden death from cardiac standstill.

Every day in the United States, as many as ten million women struggle with anorexia and bulimia. Eating disorders don't discriminate, however, and an increasing number of minority women, older women, and men are being diagnosed—children, too.

ing it as a coping mechanism to avoid or deny other negative things in their life. The overeating is usually constant but is less extreme and episodic than with binge eating disorder. Still, there are extremely serious health risks associated with this disorder, which has become an ever increasing problem in our society.

# Early Warning Signs

It's amazing how long it often takes for a parent or other family member or a friend—anyone—to notice that someone close to them has lost a significant amount of weight or is showing some other obvious signs and symptoms of an eating disorder. While people with eating disorders do get extremely good at hiding them, the signs are still very clear, even in the early stages.

The problem is that the people around the person with the eating disorder often reinforce the eating disorder behavior, at least at the start. Eating disorders often start with a weight-loss diet, and they're often accompanied by a lot of talk focused on food, weight, and appearance—especially if a partner, family member, or friend suggested the weight-loss program in the first place. This person may even participate in the dieting by becoming a partner in it—friends or family members often go on diets together. The praise for the weight loss encourages the individual to carry it even further—which will earn even more reinforcing praise at first.

Family members, friends, significant others, and spouses may originally suggest dieting because they're concerned for the individual. Sadly, obesity is especially rampant in our society. While concern for an overweight person may begin with the best of intentions, it can also create the ideal circumstances for an eating disorder to take hold. But at what point does someone who is dieting tip over into someone who's obsessively dieting and can't stop? At what point does someone who's a "picky eater" become one who binges on everything? Because they are partners in the illness at the start, it's no surprise that family members, spouses, and others are slow to realize that the weight shifts have gone too far. When the realization does hit, the person with the eating disorder suddenly starts hearing what most people would interpret as negative comments: You look too thin, you look sick, you are getting so fat. They're motivating, but in the wrong direction.

# Jolie's Story

The beginnings of the slide into anorexia are quite similar for just about all my patients.

Jolie's story is typical. She was fifteen and at a perfectly normal weight for someone her height and age—certainly not what anyone would call fat. But when Jolie went to her family doctor for a routine physical, he casually mentioned to her that she could stand to lose a few pounds. When Jolie told her mother this, she agreed. The combination of medical and parental authority convinced Jolie to go on a diet. Her mother, her father, and her friends all told her how great she looked and how they admired her willpower. Praise like that is very powerful, especially when it comes from the people who matter to you most.

The majority of people who go on a diet lose some weight and then stop dieting when they've reached—or at least neared—their goal. Jolie, however, figured that if losing a little weight was a good thing, wasn't losing a lot of weight even better? And up to a point, it was. She restricted her diet more and more and lost more and more weight. She could finally fit into those size 00 low-rise jeans—and her friends admired her for it. But something else about weight loss was even better than the praise she got. By restricting her diet so severely, Jolie actually felt better—a lot better. Why? Because underneath, Jolie was an extremely anxious individual. By focusing on the one aspect of her life that she could totally control, she was able to submerge the anxiety beneath the anorexia. Weight loss gave her life a focus that made her feel safe and in control; moreover, it also gave her a new identity.

As Jolie restricted her diet more and more, she also became more and more secretive about her eating. It took a long time for her parents to realize how thin she had become. When they did, they were horrified. The same parents who had earlier praised her for weight loss were now trying desperately to get Jolie to gain weight. They took her back to see the same doctor who had originally told her she should lose a few pounds. The doctor did the usual exam and blood tests. Jolie was very thin at that point, but medically stable. All the tests came back as normal, which meant that Jolie could say, "See, Mom, I told you I'm fine." And all the doctor said was to come back again in three months for another checkup.

Despite the normal test results, however, Jolie wasn't fine at all. Her body was in starvation mode, which meant her hormonal responses were shutting down. What's more, because starvation has powerful effects on the mind as well as the body, Jolie was now incapable of seeing herself as she really looked. Instead of seeing a near skeleton in her mirror, she saw someone overweight. At this point Jolie couldn't be reasoned with on the subject of her weight, but it was possible to get through to her on other levels. For instance, she knew that she had blacked out at school because she was so underweight and that the school administration was threatening to suspend her for medical reasons. Jolie loved school and was an excellent student. When given the choice between getting treatment and leaving school, she reluctantly agreed to see me.

I started, as I usually do, by asking Jolie to tell me what she had heard about me and why she was in my office.

"You're an eating disorder doctor. I don't have anorexia, but they're going to kick me out of school if I don't come see you twice a week and gain weight," she replied.

Jolie's response told me that she had an agenda. She would arrive exactly on time, never miss a session, and agree with everything I said. Over the next several months she would gain enough weight to reach her setpoint, not one ounce less and most definitely not one ounce more. And as soon as she gained exactly the right amount of weight and the threat of having to leave school was no longer hanging over her head, she would quit therapy. When that happened, sooner or later the eating disorder behavior would start all over again. And next time it would be harder to reverse.

I replied, "You're right, I do specialize in treating people with eating disorders, but I'm not just concerned about your weight." That really surprised Jolie. She blurted out, "But don't people with anorexia need to gain weight? Isn't that why I have to be here?"

That's when I told Jolie flat-out that I could see what her agenda was and that it wouldn't work with me: "You don't have to be in my office at all. In fact, I only want you to come back if you decide you really want to, not that you have to or because your mother or your school is making you. You have to be ready to be completely honest with me and you have to be ready to get well. I promise I'll be completely honest with you, too—and I'll do everything I can to help you get well."

Jolie was really taken aback by how quickly I had seen through her plan to be the "perfect" patient for just long enough to fool everyone into thinking she was better, and she let her guard down almost before she knew it. She thought for a moment and then said, "Sounds Okay to me. Can we talk about my weight now?"

"Not at this moment," I said. "Let's talk about school instead. What do you like best about it?" She immediately started telling me about her art class—and that gave me a glimpse into the real Jolie, the young woman whose promising artistic talent was temporarily hidden beneath the anorexia.

Later, when we started to talk more about the origin of her anorexia, Jolie told me what her doctor had said. Once again I was struck by how easily a casual remark could start the sequence of events that ended up with Jolie in my office.

# Spotting the Signs

Once you know what to look for, the early signs of eating disorder behavior become easier to spot, even though individuals with eating disorders tend to hide their behavior and their bodies, out of embarrassment and shame. In particular, they get good at convincing others that they're fine.

## Mother's Little Helper

A very common sign of anorexia is what I call "Mother's little helper." At mealtimes, the patient suddenly becomes a paragon of good daughterhood. She jumps up immediately to bring things to and from the table, then leaps up to clear the table in an instant after everyone's done eating. She's not doing this just to be helpful. She's using all that activity to distract the family from noticing how little she's eating—or from noticing that she's stuffing food into her sleeves, into her pockets, into her napkin, into the dog under the table, anywhere but her mouth. As part of her new helper role, she also now takes a deep interest in preparing food and serving it, and she's always very interested in what other people are eating. She's not doing this because she truly loves to cook, but because she's preoccupied with food, even though she's not eating much of it. An important point to remember is that people with anorexia don't lose their appetites. They're hungry all the time, although they lose hunger awareness once malnutrition sets in.

## Eating Rituals

Ritualized eating behavior is another sign of an eating disorder. Someone with an eating disorder may insist on eating only at a precisely defined time and will get frantic if the meal is served too early or too late. Another may eat only ritualized amounts—exactly nine peas or precisely two ounces of rice, for example—or only very specific foods from an

---

*Individuals with anorexia don't lose their appetites. They're hungry all the time, although they lose hunger awareness once malnutrition sets in.*

---

ever-narrowing list of possibilities. Many of my patients have used the
dietary restrictions of being a vegetarian or a vegan as a way to cover
their food restrictions. Some will spend twenty minutes cutting a piece
of food into smaller and smaller microcubes without ever actually eating
any of it.

In later stages, once the family has started to catch on, someone with
an eating disorder might insist on being left alone to eat. I had one patient who told her parents she couldn't eat with them hovering over her.
First they retreated to the kitchen while she ate alone in the dining room;
after a couple of weeks of that she made them go into their bedroom.
From there, they were banished to huddling in the garage.

## A Change in Appearance

A preoccupation with appearance, weight, and body shape is another
major sign of an eating disorder. Suddenly the individual will be very
concerned about her appearance: checking often in mirrors, stepping
on the scale many times, asking anxiously and frequently how she
looks, and worrying incessantly about her weight and her figure. She
may become very interested in ultrathin celebrities and fashion trends,
or rattle off the names of every movie star who's been in an eating disorder program. She may also start to have trouble making decisions related to her appearance. The person who once could get dressed for the
day in five minutes flat now takes an hour or longer to get ready, obsessing in front of the mirror as she tries on outfit after outfit, can't
make up her mind, and finally throws something on simply because
she's run out of time.

The clothing she does choose can be another sign of the eating disorder. At first she may select clothing that shows off—even flaunts—how
thin she is. She'll wear skimpy clothing that shows a lot of skin, or clingy
clothing that accentuates her extra-slim figure. Later on, when she has lost
virtually all her body fat, she feels cold all the time and opts for clothing
that covers her up. Conveniently, the baggy layers she's now wearing also
cover up her skeletal body in an attempt to conceal the problem, but she

can't disguise the dark circles under her eyes—a sure sign of malnutrition. To suppress the constant hunger she feels, she's suddenly chewing gum a lot and drinking lots of water, coffee, diet sodas, and diluted juices. If she starts to subsist on leafy greens and carrots instead of real food, the carotene in these vegetables can actually turn her skin a yellowish color.

## A Change in Behavior

Changes in social interaction and mood swings come with any eating disorder. Someone who once had a lot of friends and an active social life withdraws more and more, sees friends less, becomes very isolated from both friends and family. The emotional changes go way beyond typical moodiness. The individual with an eating disorder will cry frequently and get agitated easily, often over something that seems trivial. What's happening here is that severe weight fluctuations are significantly changing the brain chemistry.

In bulimia, the behavior often occurs in the evening or when no one is around—one reason why people around them may be slow to realize there's a problem. These individuals hoard food and then binge on it when they're all alone. What often happens, however, is that the next day they feel so guilty and ashamed, and so bloated and exhausted from throwing up all night, that they have a hard time getting up for school or work.

Excessive exercising can also be a sign of an eating disorder. This one, too, is fairly easy to hide at first, especially if the individual was already physically active. When the exercise goes on for hours, or when the individual now never sits still, it's likely because the exercise and fidgeting are an attempt to burn off even more calories. I'm often amazed at how patients who are so thin they should barely be able to walk can still manage to work out on a treadmill for miles. It's a good indication of how powerful the grip of an eating disorder can be.

*Mood swings occur significantly with eating disorders.*

# Getting Help

Individuals with eating disorders are usually so good at hiding them that it takes a long time for a parent, boyfriend, friend, teacher, or anyone else to finally notice. There's usually more to the situation than people simply not paying attention. Patients start out as normal teens or young adults— in fact, they often start out better than normal. The single thing I hear most often from stunned parents is "But she's such a good kid!" or "But she's never been any trouble." And that's exactly the problem. This young woman has always been good and high-achieving—got good grades, never got into trouble, always worked hard to please, never acted out, seemed to have a lot of friends, etcetera, etcetera. Parents and others have trouble associating the idea of a problem with someone who always seemed so problem-free. And quite often in the case of adolescents with eating disorders, the family is preoccupied with other problems: Another child might have a serious medical problem, or there could be a divorce in progress. Because the parents are busy with other issues, they may not notice that their good, normal, compliant child—the child they never had to worry about—is quietly and all alone falling into the depths of an eating disorder.

# Confronting the Disorder amid Mixed Messages

When someone with an eating disorder is confronted about it, the usual response is to deny that a problem exists. And they're right, in a way. For them, the eating disorder isn't a problem, it's a solution. From their perspective, they've finally found something that works for them. The eating disorder lets them escape the overwhelming anxiety that so many live with in today's society. They're not necessarily prepared to get better.

It's hard for most people to imagine how having an eating disorder could feel good. That's because most people don't suffer from the sort of severe anxiety you'd do anything, including enduring the agonies of starvation, bingeing, or purging, to relieve. Seen from that perspective, eating disorders become a lot more understandable. People who suffer from severe anxiety often never develop their own healthy identities—the anxiety gets in the way. Many of my patients don't have a clue as to who they really are. For them, an eating disorder solves two problems at once: it relieves their anxiety and gives them an identity.

Sadly, when individuals with eating disorders do seek help, the professional advice they get may not do much good. In fact, it could even make things worse. All too often, professionals are fooled and manipulated by their patients, often without realizing it. And all too many give their patients very mixed messages. One patient told me that her first therapist didn't really believe she had an eating disorder. At the initial visit, she told the patient, "You look better than I do." Needless to say, the patient very quickly realized that she could see this therapist forever without actually having to change her behavior. As an added bonus, by faithfully going to her appointments twice a week, she lulled herself, and those who cared for her, into thinking she was getting help and therefore must be getting better.

Even therapists who are savvier will often focus almost exclusively on food and weight issues. Rather than helping, this can actually make things worse. By emphasizing food and weight, they're just reinforcing the problem, by focusing the patient on the eating disorder and making the eating disorder identity even stronger. In my experience, this only makes the patient cling to her eating disorder that much more.

It's crucial—in fact, it could be a matter of life or death—to find a therapist who can truly help someone with an eating disorder. The therapist whose office is in a convenient location and who seems to be nice and sympathetic may not be the right person, unless he or she also happens to have a lot of experience with eating disorders. To find the sort of specialized help that's needed, I usually recommend contacting some of the major national eating disorder organizations and checking their referral lists to find an experienced and well-trained therapist who specializes in eating disorders.

There are definitely cases where someone who arrives at my office with an eating disorder is so medically unstable that immediate hospitalization is absolutely necessary. The neurochemical changes caused by eating disorders make it almost impossible to begin treatment until the patient is out of medical danger. That doesn't necessarily mean she has to be in a specialized eating disorder program. Any good hospital can provide the necessary medical stabilization. Once the patient is medically stable, a variety of program options for ongoing treatment can be explored: inpatient programs (IP), residential programs, transitional housing, partial hospitalization programs (PHP), day hospital programs, intensive outpatient programs (IOP), and outpatient programs (OP). Today so many patients need treatment for eating disorders that the various types of programs are available nationwide. To find one, check with national and state eating disorder organizations for referrals and program evaluations. Some of these organizations are listed in the Resources section at the back of this book.

Reaching the correct diagnosis and finding appropriate treatment for someone with an eating disorder can be difficult, frustrating, and time-consuming. The sooner the problem is acknowledged and the sooner treatment begins, the more quickly recovery can be attained. Eating disorders are complex and sometimes baffling; however, I think any eating disorder patient can find help.

# TWO

# A Diverse Disorder

*When the eating disorder* epidemic began in the 1970s, the patients who got the most media attention were young white women who came from privileged backgrounds and had anorexia or bulimia. These women were seen as a sort of entitled elite—they were already rich and now they wanted to be thin, so they chose to have an eating disorder. The media also made it seem as if getting over an eating disorder is easy. In one scene in a movie, the patient with anorexia—always a teenaged girl—is stick thin; in the next she's somehow magically cured and is eating ice cream with her therapist. Older women, men of any age, poor people, and members of minority groups were never shown. And the only eating disorders that made it into the media were anorexia and bulimia—other types of eating disorders weren't on the radar screen then.

Times have changed. Young white women from wealthier families still get eating disorders at epidemic levels, but others are catching up.

*Eating disorders are now equal opportunity: they cut across age, sex, ethnic, and income lines.*

Today about a quarter of all people diagnosed with an eating disorder are young children (as young as five), older women, or men. Members of minority groups and those with lower incomes are being diagnosed with increasing frequency. The spectrum of eating disorders has also broadened. In addition to anorexia and bulimia, more and more patients are being diagnosed with binge eating disorder and compulsive overeating.

# A Cultural Shift

As the eating disorder epidemic moves away from the standard patient stereotype, we're also experiencing a cultural shift. Our society is becoming increasingly concerned with body image and youth even as it becomes increasingly overweight and older. Television programs that emphasize the magic of cosmetic surgery make it seem as if anyone can have a designer body, while programs that focus on the glamorous lives of models and the wealthy make it appear as if having a designer body is the only desirable goal. The unconscious thinking is "If I look like that TV star or model, I'll also have her money, fame, and fabulous life." That sort of thinking is only reinforced by the proliferation of books and magazines extolling fitness and slimness and promising painless, permanent weight loss. Fashion magazines assume that being able to fit into size 00 clothing is the goal of every woman. They feature models who are clearly underweight and extol their thin figures as the perfect norm. The typical celebrity magazine or tabloid whipsaws the reader between pictures and articles about celebrities who have gotten too thin and those who have gotten too fat. They never bother to write about those who have a normal, healthy body. Similarly, the fitness magazines and many popular TV shows all feature incredibly well-toned bodies with no visible fat, telling both men and women that this is the most desirable way to look.

*The typical celebrity magazine or tabloid whipsaws the reader between pictures and articles about celebrities who have gotten too thin and those who have gotten too fat. They never bother to write about those who have a normal, healthy body.*

Everything in our society conspires to tell someone who is at a normal weight and good level of fitness that being thinner and fitter is even better—and while you're at it, looking younger is better, too. Our society tells those who are above normal weight that they are undisciplined, undeserving, and unattractive. It's no wonder that having a distorted body image is a major aspect of having an eating disorder.

## More and Younger Generations

I feel pretty secure in saying that there is also a genetic component to eating disorders. Patients or family members will often mention that a grandmother, mother, sibling, twin, aunt, cousin, or some other close relative also has an eating disorder or some form of one.

Genes alone can't account for the epidemic of eating disorders over the past decades, but at the same time, therapists are now seeing patients who represent the second or even third generation in their family to have an eating disorder. Even without the genetic component, the family environment has a huge influence. If the family is very preoccupied and concerned with food, weight, and appearance, they can pass this concern on to their kids. I've had patients as young as five tell me how worried they are about eating the "wrong" foods and getting fat. Children who grow up seeing constant dieting, constant concern about weight, and constant working out absorb the messages that food is the enemy and appearance is all.

# Elizabeth's Story

I never thought someone as young as five could end up in my office until I met Elizabeth. How do you treat a child with an eating disorder?

Even at the age of five, Elizabeth was an extremely perceptive child. She was very aware of her mother's dieting behavior and constant concern with food, weight, and appearance. I had learned early on that children with eating disorders are unable to separate their own identities from their parents' identities. Because her mother was always on a diet and worrying about her weight, Elizabeth assumed she needed to shadow her mother's behavior. Imitating the person most important to her, she began constantly judging her body and restricting her food. This quickly spiraled into an eating disorder that was out of control.

I knew from my preadolescent and adolescent patients that parents can assist in their child's recovery by becoming teachers by example. I decided to use this same approach with Elizabeth and her mother. In our sessions, I worked with Elizabeth to develop her sense of an independent self and help her realize that children don't have to be little grown-ups mimicking everything their parents do. At the same time, I worked with her mother on changing the damaging messages about food and appearance she was sending to her child. In the end, both Elizabeth and her mother had a better sense of themselves. I continued to see them both for several years. When Elizabeth was about fifteen, I met with her and her mother again. Both of them later wrote to me about their experience.

## Words from Elizabeth

At the time my eating disorder started, I was afraid to get help, because I was unsure of what that meant. I realized that having an eating disorder was hurting the people around me and myself. I didn't want to hurt the people around me or myself any longer.

I realized that my life was spinning out of control. I thought I was going to die and couldn't focus anymore. I was eating little pieces of paper to fill the void of food and running circles in my room every day to burn off the thoughts that filled my head.

The eating disorder identity became unsafe to own any longer and also became deadly. Others ask me, What made you finally decide to leave the eating disorder identity? I tell them the reasons were my family's support and wanting a second chance on life.

Through therapy I learned that to reclaim recovery I needed something else to replace the eating disorder. My love for horses became one of the answers. I was able to use equine therapy, which taught me how to take care of a horse and gave me a reason to become stronger to learn to ride it. Through the process of therapy I learned that grooming and feeding the horse at the stables was a form of care. I was able to transfer the lesson of care onto myself and found my second chance of life.

I no longer have the perspective of a child, but now the perspective of a young adult. I know that perfect doesn't exist. Nobody is perfect; we all have our flaws and we can't possibly change them all. I know even when I have my good days and bad days that I cannot choose a life dictated by an eating disorder any longer.

## Words from Elizabeth's Mother

After going through this experience with Elizabeth, I can speak from the heart. I tell parents to be aware of what is going on in their child's life and watch the messages that they give to their children. They are so fragile, and what parents say and how they act may reinforce negative thinking.

Initially I never realized my comments had such an impact on Elizabeth. I could get depressed about it, or I could learn from my own experiences. I had the constant thought that if I stayed in the guilt, how was I going to help her?

I learned that parents need to go through their own healing process. They need to find the help that best matches their own needs as well as their children's.

We are still learning as a whole family and still making mistakes, but now there is an awareness and a sensitivity level for continuous healing.

In effect, the messages from the family and the outside world are setting these kids up for an eating disorder. Unfortunately, eating disorders affect people of all ages, even the innocent child.

# Eating Disorders in Midlife

The emphasis on youth in our society puts a lot of pressure on women at midlife. The women their age they see in the media all look very fit, slender, and youthful. Of course, the youthful, trim appearance of many celebrities is artificial. It's the result of cosmetic surgery, liposuction, personal trainers, and strict dieting that approaches—if it hasn't reached—the level of an eating disorder. To fit into her teenaged daughter's clothing, a typical woman at midlife will need to do the same things, including have the eating disorder.

These women with eating disorders are typically not relapsing back into an illness they had when they were younger. Most of them have no previous history and develop their disorder as mature adults, often over the age of forty. They're usually married with children. In almost every case, they're now facing a time of major transition in their lives. For many, their role as a mother is changing as their children grow up and leave home. Some are also finding that their role as a wife is changing as they face divorce or the death of a husband.

Many of the women at midlife who come to me for treatment are well

*The underlying issues of anxiety, obsessiveness, and perfectionism don't change with age.*

educated and have had successful careers before they decided to become full-time wives and mothers. That role as family caretaker was one they understood, and it fit well with their personalities. The problem comes when the family changes and the caretaker role isn't needed as much. Suddenly there's a lot of empty time and a feeling of not being valued anymore, and this may coincide with concerns about appearance.

Not every older woman with an eating disorder is a stay-at-home mom now suffering from empty-nest syndrome. A number of my patients have families and also successful careers. They, too, have difficulty with societal pressures and family changes, plus they have to deal with the transitions and frustrations of their working life. Many come into therapy feeling that they were somehow, a long time ago, diverted away from the things that really interested them and into career tracks that are wrong for them. They'd like to go back and do the things they always wanted to do but never got support for, but at the same time they feel they're too old to make major career changes. The incidence of eating disorders is rising very rapidly in this age group, to the point where there are now residential and day programs designed specifically for women at midlife.

As with any patients, women at midlife sometimes enter treatment voluntarily when they recognize for themselves that a big problem has developed. Others need to be pushed into treatment. Many of my patients are brought in by spouses or referred to me by other therapists, physicians, friends, and even personal trainers. Sometimes it's the children who recognize an eating disorder in their mother. I walked out of my office into my waiting room one afternoon several years ago and found a young man named Sam asking for me. He didn't have an appointment, but he was desperate to talk with me. I told him we could chat at the end of the day, when I had seen all my other patients. He waited patiently for me for nearly five hours. When I could finally sit down with him, Sam told me immediately that his mother had had an eating disorder for several years but was still basically healthy. He would be leaving for college soon, and he was very worried that his departure would make her illness worse. He wanted me to agree to treat her. I was very touched by his concern and felt his mother needed help, but she would have to be the one to initiate the treatment. I don't know what Sam said to her, but she called the next week.

The underlying issues of anxiety, obsessiveness, and perfectionism don't change with age. I treat women at midlife in exactly the same way as all my patients, by establishing a trust relationship with them. That can be very difficult. These women have been in charge of busy households for years, and they're not accustomed to being vulnerable and revealing themselves. They also find it hard to rediscover their old passions and find healthy ways to redirect their energy. They feel they're too old and too out of touch with the job market to begin significant new careers. They have a point. Age and sex discrimination may be illegal, but they exist nonetheless, and it is difficult to find jobs that are appropriate for their age and education level. Some patients solve this problem by going back to school to pursue a passion. Several of my patients have become chefs or professors, for example, and a number have gone back to pursue graduate work. Many have used their experience in volunteer work and their extensive social networks to find satisfying volunteer jobs in areas outside their previous world of schools and children.

# Natalie's Story

Empty-nest syndrome—the idea that a mother loses her self when her children grow up and leave home—may seem like a cliché, but there's a strong basis of truth in it. Not every mother has a hard time with this transition, but it can be a major trigger for developing an eating disorder. The case of Natalie is a classic example.

Natalie was fifty-four years old when she entered therapy for severe anorexia. Although she had no previous history of an eating disorder, Natalie had many of the personality traits that often go along with the illness. In particular, she was a strong perfectionist. Before her marriage, Natalie had earned an MBA from a prestigious program and had worked as a management consultant. She married, soon had a child, and left the workforce for good. Raising her four children with little help from her workaholic husband gave Natalie plenty of room to use her management skills—and her perfectionism. She became very active in her children's schools and after-school programs.

But when Natalie's children left home for college, she was home alone with little to occupy her time and no financial need to return to work. Her identity had been closely tied to her role as a mother. Now that her children were independent, Natalie needed a new identity. She discovered it by accident when she became interested in organic foods. The idea of healthier eating soon became an increasing preoccupation with eating the "right" foods. In moderation this is a good thing, but in Natalie's case it became orthorexia—an excessive concern about eating healthier. Her food preoccupation went far beyond eating only organically grown foods. She began eliminating all foods that didn't fit into her rigid idea of healthy eating. That led to restricting her diet more and more, which in turn led to weight loss. During this time Natalie became menopausal, a time when women normally begin to lose some bone mass. Her doctor advised her to do more weight-bearing exercise as a way to slow the loss. Natalie took this advice to an extreme and added overexercising on a treadmill to her orthorexia.

At first, Natalie's husband and friends were very supportive of her decision to eat better, and they approved of the weight loss recommended by her doctor and family. The reinforcement she got led her to be even more involved in orthorexia and exercising. Her diet grew more and more restricted, her eating became more and more ritualistic, and she was exercising several hours a day. Rather than making her healthier, however, this obsessive concern about food was making her sicker, with fatigue, mood swings, and digestive problems. Her orthorexia had evolved into anorexia.

Natalie couldn't understand why she was eating "healthy" but feeling worse. Her physician checked her out carefully for serious illness such as stomach cancer and found nothing. Based on Natalie's description of how she was now spending her days, he referred her to a psychiatrist, who referred her to me, as a specialist in eating disorders.

In our sessions Natalie told me how empty she felt her life was now that her children didn't need her. She regretted that she had given up her career and felt she had wasted her life. Menopause made her feel less desirable as a woman, even though her relationship with her husband had actually become closer now that the house was empty and they had more time for each other. He still wasn't home much, though, and despite a wide network of acquaintances in her community Natalie was extremely lonely. All the passion, energy, and perfectionism that she had once poured into raising her family now had nowhere to go except back onto Natalie herself.

As we talked, it became clear that many of Natalie's ideas about good nutrition and safe levels of exercise had been picked up in fragments from TV shows and health magazines. In therapy, we focused not on what she was eating, but on how she felt. Natalie realized that she was trying to fill the terrible inner emptiness she felt. She needed to make a transition from being a very involved mother into being something else—something healthier than having an eating disorder.

Natalie felt that her MBA skills were too rusty to look for another job in management. What she did have, however, was years of experience as a volunteer in school-related activities. When we talked more about those years, Natalie realized that the volunteer work she had enjoyed most was in an after-school reading program.

It took several months of therapy before Natalie felt physically and mentally strong enough to act on her interest. She approached the school administrator in charge of the reading program and asked if she could volunteer again. The administrator was delighted to have such a well-educated and experienced volunteer.

Natalie still eats organic foods, along with other kinds of food, and she still spends time on her treadmill, but she now limits the amount of exercise time. She finds the volunteer work very satisfying and thrives in the structured environment it provides.

# Men with Eating Disorders

The number of men with eating disorders has skyrocketed in recent years. As with women at midlife, today there are programs designed only for men with eating disorders—but on a limited basis.

Men, especially young men in their teens and twenties, face tremendous societal pressure to be muscular and toned, with six-pack abs and bulging biceps. Older men face societal pressure to look youthful, although our culture doesn't put the same emphasis on this for men as it does for women—yet. To look the way the male models in fitness magazines look requires a strict diet and hours in the gym each day, to say nothing of cosmetic surgery, but most people don't realize that. Many of the male patients I see have ended up with eating disorders that started out as a way to look more like the buffed-out images they see in the media, or they weren't secure in their gender identity.

For many men, the body image issue arises when they are in their teens. Sports can increase concern for body image, because they put a premium on strong, well-developed muscles, fitness, and little body fat. Some sports, such as wrestling, track, and gymnastics, stress being as light and strong as possible and encourage participants to "cut" weight.

Excessive concern for body image doesn't have to start with sports, however. For many young men it starts as an attempt to improve their appearance and self-confidence through weight loss and muscle development. Dieting—often in a very unhealthy and distorted way—along with weight training and exercise are the usual methods. For individuals who already tend toward anxiety and perfectionism, discovering bodybuilding and the dieting that goes with it can have a special appeal. They can become obsessive about their training, following very restrictive diets and taking a lot of natural supplements that are supposed to help build

---

*Older men face societal pressure to look youthful, although our culture doesn't put the same emphasis on this for men as it does for women—yet.*

*Men with eating disorders are still a hidden population. Despite the increasing attention eating disorders get, the number of men who enter into treatment is small and probably considerably below the number who need it.*

muscle and endurance. Among serious bodybuilders and other athletes, vomiting from exercising after eating is not uncommon. It's not usually deliberate, but it is accepted as something that can occasionally happen as part of training. So is skipping a meal or restricting intake before a workout, practice session, or competition. That level of acceptance makes it even easier for someone who is training obsessively to step over the line into an eating disorder.

Someone who begins to work out and watch his diet gets a lot of reinforcement and praise for deciding to shape up. The positive effects of weight training can be seen within a few weeks—most young men can build muscle quickly if they train regularly—and that leads to a lot more positive feedback. As he packs on the muscle, a young man will probably gain weight even though he's restricting his diet. For a vulnerable individual, that can start the loop of more training and less eating. He looks better and weighs more, not less, but at this point his physical appearance is masking an eating disorder. One of my patients was beginning his second year as a law student at an Ivy League school when he began working out and dieting as a way to relieve stress and look good for job interviews. He quickly got sucked into a cycle of exercise bulimia, but he was able to hide the symptoms so well behind his bigger muscles, fit appearance, and slight weight gain that nobody noticed—until he collapsed in the gym late in the spring. He was forced to take a medical leave and didn't return for two years.

For some men, confusion about their sexuality or gender identity can lead to an eating disorder. Many get interested in weight loss and body building as a way to conform more to a physical image of masculinity, and then discover that dieting and overexercising help relieve some of the tremendous anxiety sex or gender issues are causing. From there it's just a short step to an eating disorder.

## Jerome's Story

Jerome was an outwardly successful plastic surgeon with a prospering practice. He came to see me because he could nip and tuck everyone but himself.

A Latino from a poor family, Jerome had always found it difficult to have his own identity. He was a good student and a talented musician with a strong perfectionist personality. He had gone to a performing arts high school instead of his neighborhood school and to college on a music scholarship. In college, his interests changed suddenly, and he switched over to a very competitive premed program. He was accepted to a top medical school and went on to become a top plastic surgeon—a process that took years of very hard work and dedication. As well, while he was in medical school, Jerome came out as a gay man.

Jerome had felt driven to overachieve ever since grade school. For all his successes, he always felt hollow inside, as if someone else was getting all the good grades, awards, and professional advancement. Jerome thought that his endless anxiety and the nagging sense of himself as a fraud and a failure would go away once he acknowledged his sexuality. That wasn't really the problem, however—as with most people who have an eating disorder, the true issues were anxiety and perfectionism. As Jerome achieved more and more professional competence and success, he felt less and less that he had a real identity. At times he felt he was only wearing the mask of a doctor; he was also still very uncertain about his sexual identity. Because he was a plastic surgeon, he was also spending his days dealing with people who were very concerned with their body image. Not surprisingly, some of that concern rubbed off on Jerome. He grew increasingly dissatisfied with his own body.

He began smothering his anxiety by becoming preoccupied with food and weight loss. His eating patterns became very disordered, and his weight would fluctuate up and down. Jerome never developed all the defining symptoms of bulimia or anorexia, so his diagnosis was put down as eating disorder not otherwise specified—even in his eating disorder, Jerome had a conflict of identity. He realized that he had to stop the disordered eating before it developed into something worse and began to interfere with his professional life. We're working together now to help Jerome define himself better as a person and learn to cope better with his anxiety. His disordered eating is definitely improving. It's still a problem, but Jerome feels more in control now and better able to resist the temptation to hide within the disorder.

# Ethnic Changes

In recent years, the ethnic mix of my patients has become much broader. I now see many more patients whose heritage is African-American, Hispanic, Asian, or some other ethnicity. Many are young women who come from somewhat closed religious or immigrant communities. There's a lot of pressure on these women to maintain a particular appearance and conform to family and community expectations. The high incidence of eating disorders within these communities is a silent epidemic. Families try to keep the problem hushed up and out of public view for fear of embarrassment.

In some communities, particularly the African-American community, women are cautious about being too thin. Even so, it's easy to see the societal norm for the pressure to be thin in all ethnic backgrounds.

Westernized concepts of attractiveness in a woman can be at real odds with the community concept. I recently had a patient who had come to the United States a couple of years before to do graduate work. She didn't start out thinking of herself as overweight, but she quickly fell into the American body image/weight trap and became severely anorexic.

As she told me in treatment, "In my country, the concept of beauty is intelligence. Here, beauty is all about appearance."

# THREE

# Illusions of Perfection

*Anxiety.* It's a fundamental issue among individuals with eating disorders. Suffering from overpowering but undefined feelings of dread and agitation, a constant, overwhelming sense that something bad is about to happen—*internal anxiety*—the person with an eating disorder will become preoccupied with how the outside world views her, which in turn provokes a feeling of *external anxiety.* Constant reassurance and approval is sought to ease the external anxiety. How can you be sure of getting constant reassurance and outside approval? One way is to channel all that anxiety into being perfect. And one way to be perfect is to eat perfectly.

Many people with eating disorders have found that controlling their eating can seem like the answer to the search for relief from anxiety and for perfection. They can create rigid rules for themselves and actually stick to them. They can engage in ritualistic behavior and see it pay off as they lose weight. Until their weight loss becomes frightening, they can continue to get the approval and respect of others. And because they control what they eat, they feel in control of their anxiety—at least for a time.

# The Allure of Perfectionism

Perfectionism—a powerful, sometimes irrational, urge to do everything exactly right—is a personality trait that's very common among people with eating disorders. Perfectionists impose impossibly high, completely unrealistic demands on themselves. It's a way of trying to deal with severe anxiety. By the reasoning of the perfectionist, controlling everything in life can help prevent the supposed bad things from happening. Perfectionism is almost always an attempt to get all that anxiety under control and keep it that way.

Perfectionism isn't necessarily a bad thing—in moderation. It's the strong desire to do your best and reach a high level of accomplishment that keeps talented musicians practicing, talented athletes training, and talented artists creating. But for many people, perfectionism isn't really connected to a sense of accomplishment and achievement. Their anxiety levels are so acutely high that no accomplishment is ever good enough, and striving to achieve just leads to further anxiety. Rather than giving them control over their anxiety and their lives, perfectionism actually spins these individuals even more out of control and deeper into unbearable anxiety. When a desperately anxious person with an *obsessive identity* discovers that the one thing that can be completely controlled is what gets put into the body, what you have is a perfectionist with an eating disorder.

---

*Perfectionists impose impossibly high demands on themselves. It's a way of trying to deal with severe anxiety. Unfortunately, striving to achieve may lead to further anxiety, to the point that it becomes unbearable.*

---

# The Roots of Perfectionism

Not everyone who has to deal with a lot of anxiety copes with it by developing an eating disorder. I can't say for sure why some people feel anxiety so much more acutely than others, but I do think genetics is a factor. As a therapist I can often detect signs of perfectionism or obsessive-compulsive disorder in a parent or other family member—a clue that the patient may also have the problem.

Genes alone, however, won't make you a perfectionist. How you're raised plays a big role. Young children depend on the approval of others—parents especially—to develop their own sense of self. Eventually, as kids get older and enter adolescence, they begin to learn to value themselves for themselves, and not always to depend on the approval of others for their self-esteem. Some, though, have trouble getting past the external standards of others. Because they have difficulty developing their own internal standards, they continue to look outward and to rely on others for validation. If family members, friends, and others also have high expectations for them, the problem of perfection can get even worse. The praise of others ends up being more important to them than any internal sense of accomplishment they might feel, and in fact, they often don't feel any real satisfaction at all.

---

Perfectionists with eating disorders have their own grading scale. Listed below are the ultimate ideals.

A = Anorexia

B = Bulimia/Binge eating

C = Compulsive overeating

D = Dieting and Exercise

F = Fat failure

# The Perfectionist Child

Perfectionists need to control their own world. Their basic personality makes them very sensitive to the anxiety of daily living, and control over at least some aspects of life helps them cope. The tendency toward perfectionism often shows up early. These are the children who not only put their toys away without being told but put them away in size order.

When you're a perfectionist personality, childhood works for you really well, because it is concrete and simple. Behaviors are either good or bad, and good behavior usually leads to clear rewards. If you're good at the doctor's office, you get a lollipop; if you're good in the classroom, you get a gold star. As a child, you quickly learn that you can master your small universe by doing well in school, by being nice to your parents, by making a good impression on authority figures. Do all those things, and the rewards of approval automatically follow.

Once you hit adolescence, though, your universe becomes larger and a lot harder to control. Puberty makes your body change rapidly, and that's something you can't control at all. You're having all sorts of new thoughts about things like sex—thoughts that can be very confusing. At the same time, you're expected to start thinking in a more mature, abstract way, to be more responsible, and to rely less on external approval. If you're a concrete, things-are-either-black-or-white sort of person, these changes can be very difficult to adjust to. In today's society, there's an added issue for girls: They're entering puberty at a much younger age, not at twelve or thirteen, as was once the norm, but at ten or sometimes even younger. The emotional development of these girls is not aligned with their physiology. They have the bodies of more mature young women but the minds of children, and that can be very confusing.

Perfectionist adolescents find that the relatively controlled world they created for themselves as children doesn't exist anymore. That creates a lot of anxiety—and the way a perfectionist copes with anxiety is by becoming even more concrete and focused on the control of external things.

As these kids grow older, they're the ones who keep their rooms perfectly neat, do perfectly well on their schoolwork, behave perfectly to their parents and teachers, and otherwise seem to be great, problem-free kids. Because they seem to be such great kids, they can have a severe eating disorder yet still stay under the crisis radar in their families for a really long time. What parent wouldn't be happy to have a child who always does homework without being nagged? Who's organized, who's never the subject of a worried parent-teacher conference? Who does really well at some activity like gymnastics or the yearbook? Okay, maybe you do have to spend a lot of time calming the kid down and being reassuring, but that's a good sort of problem, right? I've had plenty of parents look at their kid's messy room, underachieving schoolwork, and challenging behavior and ask me half-jokingly if there's a way to give their child a dose of perfectionism. I always tell them their child is already perfect—a perfectly normal teenager.

It's the perfectionist child who's at the highest risk for developing an eating disorder as a teenager or young adult. In childhood, when life was simpler, the anxiety could be controlled. Now the only way to control the anxiety is with obsessive behaviors that become increasingly dysfunctional, to the point of taking over the individual's identity. Once adulthood enters the picture, the obsessive identity is full of the internal and external anxiety that increases perfectionism. The goals that perfectionists strive for as children, adolescents, and ultimately adults are the same: they're always organized, always praised, always liked, always taking care of others, always juggling multitudes of activities and responsibilities, always overachieving—and always anxious.

*Perfectionist adolescents find that the relatively controlled world they created for themselves as children doesn't exist anymore. That creates a lot of anxiety.*

# Self-Defeating Behavior

Perfectionism as a way to control anxiety doesn't work very well. All it really does is raise a whole new set of problems that have to be solved by more perfectionism. On the surface, that might seem like a good thing: One way of being a perfectionist is to work really hard to be the best. That sort of thinking can lead to very high levels of genuine accomplishment. The problem is that these individuals feel they can never perfectly achieve enough. Their perfectionism is unrelenting and ultimately becomes self-defeating. Their brain says, "Reach this destination and you'll be perfect," but then, when the goal is attained, their brain resets the destination to something further out of reach. They can never get to the goal, because they can never get past the process of attaining perfection. The process, not the end product, can become the real focus of activity.

## Rules and Rituals

One of my patients, Lexi, is a talented artist, but before she can get down to work on a painting, everything around her has to be perfect. The house has to be perfectly clean and completely organized. Lexi's closet is a work of art in itself. Everything in it is arranged perfectly by color, like a rainbow. Everything within each color is arranged by category. Among the white clothing, for instance, all the shirts are together: first the long-sleeved shirts, followed by the short-sleeved shirts, followed by the sleeveless shirts. Lexi takes the same approach to her studio. Before she can start work, it has to be perfectly clean and her work materials have to be organized in exactly the right way. Then, and only then, can she begin a painting. The problem is that by the time she's cleaned and organized the house and her studio, a good part of the day has gone by and she's exhausted. It doesn't leave much time for actual painting.

*Perfectionists can never get to the goal because they can never get past the process of attaining perfection. The process, not the product, becomes the real focus of activity.*

When she does get down to painting, Lexi is incredibly self-critical. She'll throw away something it took days to make because it doesn't meet her standard of perfection. She won't allow anyone to see her work in progress. She'll show her art only if she's convinced it is perfect and totally complete. Despite the many, many hours Lexi spends on her art, her standard of perfection for herself is so impossibly high that she has little to show for it.

As Lexi's situation shows, getting trapped in the perfection process often leads to more self-defeating behavior. Perfectionists can end up in an endless cycle of highly ritualized activity. They create strict rules for themselves, thinking that if they follow those rules to the letter they won't make any mistakes. Perfectionists cage themselves in with a rigid set of behaviors. They inevitably break their own unrealistic rules, which leads to further feelings of guilt and failure, which leads to further anxiety, which leads to more rituals and rules, which leads to . . . you get the idea. Their constant "failures" lead perfectionists to become extremely self-critical and self-blaming.

## Procrastination

Major procrastination is very common among perfectionists. Because they're afraid they won't live up to their own high standards and the standards they think others expect of them, they often put off doing something important for as long as possible. They think they're trying to figure out exactly the right way to do the work—and they assume that there's one and only one exactly right approach. That leads to

---

*Perfectionism can lead to behavior that can seriously interfere with normal life.*

---

procrastination, often by focusing on irrelevant or minor details of the project. When the absolute last minute finally arrives, they'll go into a whirlwind of activity and get the job done. I've seen this time and time again with my patients: they put off that term paper or important professional presentation until the night before and then work nonstop to get it done.

I had one patient, a young man named Paul, whose perfectionism and procrastination cost him several good jobs. Paul had graduated from a prestigious college with a business degree. When applying for jobs, he always did well on the interview and would get the offer. Things would start off well, but then Paul's perfectionism would kick in. He'd put off getting down to the real work of a project, instead spending hours getting organized to get started. He'd organize himself to the point of paralysis—actually doing the work would disrupt his elaborately crafted organizational plan. His anxiety level would rise and rise as he found himself frozen and unable to get the project under way. As the deadline neared, Paul would end up taking a lot of work home with him and staying up all night working on it in a frenzy. He'd be late for work the next day, or he'd come in on time but be so tired he couldn't stay awake in meetings. He'd also be so tired or so caught up in work that he'd cancel his appointments with me at the last minute or just not show up at all. In the end, Paul's projects were always completed on time and done extremely well, but the process of getting to the outstanding end product was very hard for him and disruptive for the company. Paul would eventually be let go.

Some perfectionists so fear failure that their procrastination gets worse over time, sometimes to the point of reaching a sort of paralysis. Rather than try something and come up short of their own impossibly high standard, they end up not trying at all.

*Procrastination is both an expression of anxiety and
something that makes anxiety worse.*

Most of us procrastinate now and then, of course, and most of us have pulled the occasional all-nighter to get a term paper or work report finished, but that's very different from the constant procrastination combined with high anxiety that are major aspects of perfectionism. That's a bad combination, because eventually you'll do almost anything to reduce the anxiety level. To avoid having to procrastinate and be anxious about doing a term paper, for instance, you might decide to just drop out of school altogether. Your sense of yourself as a constant failure makes that choice even easier.

## Excessive Activity

The flip side of perfectionist procrastination is excessive activity. Rather than put off that important report to the last night, a perfectionist might work on it obsessively for days, endlessly tweaking details, trying to make it exactly right—and, of course, worrying about it the entire time. I once had a patient named Brenda who was constantly working very hard on her college term papers, to the point where she had little time to do anything else. She'd start each paper the very day it was assigned and work on it endlessly. With every paper, at some point she would get obsessed with some minor aspect and spend days pursuing it, tracking down obscure research and reading material that wasn't really relevant to the main topic. Once she got down to actually writing the paper, she would go through a dozen drafts before she was satisfied. For all the huge amounts of work that went into each paper, she still always handed them in late.

## The All-or-Nothing Mind-Set

Perfectionists end up seeing things in very concrete, all-or-nothing terms: For example, a B+ instead of an A+ on a test is the same as total failure. And if you're the sort of person who thinks in such black-and-white terms, you might decide that getting a B+ means you're doomed to a lifetime of inadequacy. You might then take that thinking to the next step, which is to decide that it's better to just give up on getting good grades completely, since you'll obviously never get an A on anything ever again. Similarly, the mildest criticism or even a friendly suggestion for improvement from a boss could send you into a panic over being fired—and you might decide to quit instead.

*While perfectionism* can lead to high accomplishment, it can also lead in the opposite direction, to a lot of really negative things, such as school phobia, social anxiety disorder, separation anxiety, isolation, and burnout. The perfectionist might be the perfect friend, all supportive and helpful—or she might be the perfect evil bitch, bullying those around her. The perfectionist model often works in the negative. The mind of a perfectionist is constantly saying, "You'll never be good enough." I've had patients who have required immediate inpatient treatment for weight stabilization tell me that their bodies aren't thin enough to be perfect.

Perfectionists will judge their body image by the more unrealistic standards set by the society around us. These demands for perfection are unrealistic and virtually impossible to achieve. They're formed not by

---

*Perfectionists will judge their body image by the more unrealistic standards set by the society around us, by the endless media images of so-called perfect bodies that bombard us every day.*

---

the reality of what a healthy body should look like but by the endless media images of so-called perfect bodies that bombard us every day. That sort of perfection isn't really something any normal person can attain without major body-altering means such as extremely strenuous exercise, starvation dieting, and cosmetic surgery, but the images are still very, very powerful. Combine our societal pressure to be slender with a perfectionist's drive to be perfect, and what you get is someone who will be very vulnerable to a major eating disorder.

In addition to setting unrealistic goals for herself, typically someone who's a perfectionist will set unrealistic goals for others and will expect levels of performance that will always be disappointing. Seeking perfection in everyone and everything, the perfectionist is bound to be disappointed. Moreover, when other people come up short, the perfectionist is likely to label them a failure and perhaps even reject them.

The anxiety perfectionists experience when they don't meet the expectations of those around them can send them into a real tailspin. They just failed at the thing they thought they were best at. What's left? Not much, because their obsessive identity until now has been totally tied to being perfect. The solution is to find something else to be perfect at, something that they can do better than anyone else, something that they can completely control.

Unfortunately, the perfectionism that leads someone to have the early signs of an eating disorder also lets her persist with it. As anyone who's ever gone on a weight-loss diet knows, it's very hard to limit your intake of food and feel hungry all the time. You'll probably give up within a few weeks. However, if you've got an obsessive identity, you'll be able to stick with your self-imposed restrictions and even make them stricter as time goes by. As you restrict more and more, the same

---

*Seeking perfection in everyone and everything, the
perfectionist is bound to be disappointed.*

---

perfectionism that got you started on the eating disorder path is only re-inforced by the physiological changes that starvation from the eating disorder causes in the brain. We know from many studies that individuals with eating disorders develop powerful obsessive-compulsive thoughts and behavior.

# Emma's Story

I've been treating Emma for anorexia for a couple of years. She's one of the most perfectionistic patients I've ever had.

Outwardly, Emma seems like a healthy, normal, happy individual. Inwardly, she's filled with shame and a strong sense of inadequacy. The origins of those feelings took a long time to come out—we were many sessions into therapy—but when they did, they explained a lot. Emma was a bright but very anxious child, eager to learn but also easily distracted by her anxiety. In first grade, her perfectionist tendencies and high anxiety level led to her diagnosis as learning disabled. In front of the whole class, Emma's teacher called out her name and told her she was being sent to the resource room, the place where the "special" students went. Suddenly Emma was isolated from her classmates and labeled with a new identity: stupid. But Emma knew she wasn't stupid, and her new identity left her feeling confused and even more anxious. She felt like an outcast and soon started acting like one, helped along by her perfectionism. She isolated herself from other kids, had trouble making friends, couldn't establish good relations with her teachers, and stopped trusting anyone.

Emma sought out a new label. In sixth grade, she befriended an outcast with the label "fat." Emma was soon mimicking her friend's ritualized dieting behavior, and she discovered a new label: anorexia. Here was an identity ideal for Emma, one that gave her perfectionism a focus and finally helped her manage all that anxiety. From that point onward, Emma's mind told her never to eat more one day than she had the day before. Her weight plummeted, but her schoolwork began to thrive. Emma had found a way to channel the anxiety that had kept her from learning easily when she was younger. Now her true intelligence could shine and she could put all that perfectionism to use. Not only could she shed the stupid label, she could show everyone how wrong it had been—and she received huge amounts of praise for "overcoming" her "disability." Emma did well in high school, yet her only memories of that time were of feeling tremendous anxiety and inadequacy.

In college, Emma continued to do well academically, but her eating disorder was becoming even more serious. She was now restricting her intake during the day, while bingeing and purging in the evenings. In between, she would run for miles as a way of numbing her inner turmoil. She thought she was in complete control, but she also felt separate, extremely alone, and different from anyone else. She gradually became more and more obsessed with food and exercise, to the point where her thoughts about how to plan the perfect day of perfect eating and perfect running kept her awake most of the night.

The neurochemical changes of near-starvation led to anxiety, mood swings, and even more obsessive thinking. She was so obsessed with food and exercise that she barely noticed that she had also become severely depressed. When disabling panic attacks set in, however, Emma finally realized that she was no longer in control of anything. Her anxiety and her perfectionism had created an obsessive identity—and it was that powerful false identity that was now in charge.

Emma had to withdraw from college for over a year to regain her self, in part through an admission to a residential eating disorder program. She was able to return to school, graduate with honors, and begin her career in marketing. Despite all these successes, underneath she still often feels that she's a failure who will never be good enough, no matter how hard she works. Her own identity, however, is now strong enough that she can handle the stresses of her job without being tempted to fall back into the obsessive identity.

# The Obsessive Identity

The idea of the obsessive identity got me thinking about other psychological problems that were deeply rooted in anxiety. When I was running an adolescent medicine division, I saw many young patients whose psychological problems were also deeply rooted in anxiety and identity issues, but who didn't have eating disorders. What many of them did have was obsessive-compulsive disorder. And the more I dealt with patients who had eating disorders, the more I realized that they had a lot in common with OCD patients. In fact, I started to realize that many, though not all, individuals with eating disorders had an obsessive identity. Their eating disorder, rooted in their obsessive behavior, had become their sense of self, to the exclusion of anything else. And with that insight, eating disorders suddenly were a lot less baffling. Now I had a framework for understanding the roots of the problem.

## The Obsessive Identity

*These independent components (perfectionism, anxiety, and OCD)*
*work together to produce the obsessive identity, which is*
*a core component of the eating disorder identity.*

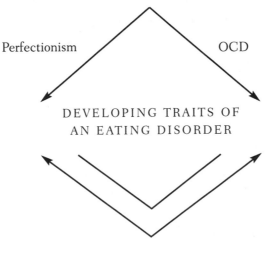

Perfectionism          OCD

DEVELOPING TRAITS OF
AN EATING DISORDER

Internal and External Anxiety

Anxiety and the drive to perfectionism are closely linked to obsessive-compulsive disorder. People with OCD show a lot of ritualistic, repetitive behaviors that interfere with everyday functioning. When OCD, anxiety, and perfectionism come together in a vulnerable individual—particularly someone who doesn't have a strong identity—all the ingredients for obsessive behavior about food and eating are in place. This interrelated diagnostic triad is at the core of many eating disorders.

I really prefer not to label my patients with the OCD diagnosis. Labels are very limiting, and they tend to blind people to other aspects of the situation. Instead, I like to define OCD in another way: *Overwhelming Controlling Desire*. In many ways I see this as a better description of the obsessive identity that is so common among people with eating disorders. They have a desperate desire to control the overwhelming internal and external anxiety that fills their lives.

## Obsessive-Compulsive Disorder (OCD)

Today we're all much more aware of obsessive-compulsive disorder as a serious psychological problem. Despite that, there are still a lot of misconceptions about exactly what OCD means. To understand the connection between anxiety, OCD, and eating disorders, we need to be as exact as possible.

Let's start with the obsessive part of the disorder. People with OCD have obsessive thoughts, impulses, or mental images that are inappropriate and intrusive. The thoughts cause severe anxiety or distress, mostly because they're not just excessive worry about real-life problems. For most people with OCD, the obsessions aren't usually even related to any actual real-life problem. Someone with OCD might worry excessively about whether a door is locked, for instance, and will constantly check and recheck to make sure it is.

Another aspect of OCD is that the person tries to ignore the obsessive thoughts or neutralize them by some other thought or action. Trying to ignore obsessive thoughts altogether or forcing yourself to think of something else is very difficult and creates a great deal of anxiety.

Obsessions lead to compulsive and repetitive behaviors, such as washing

---

*Compulsions are repetitive behaviors with rules that have
to be rigidly followed, usually in response to anxiety
or obsession.*

---

your hands over and over or constantly checking to be sure the oven is turned off, or repetitive mental acts, such as praying or counting, that someone feels driven to perform. Most of the time these acts have rules that must be rigidly followed. So someone with an obsession about germs might compulsively wash her hands over and over again, always in a very particular way. Anything that disrupts that routine would be very upsetting.

For people with OCD, the whole point of all the ritualized behavior and thinking is to relieve anxiety or keep some awful thing from happening. The OCD behavior, however, isn't realistically connected with the thing it's trying to prevent. In the case of a germ obsession, compulsive hand washing is performed supposedly to avoid getting sick. Because hand washing does help prevent illness, there's a basis in reality to the compulsion. But someone with OCD might wash her hands ten times in a row every time she returns home, and be convinced that if she doesn't do it this exact way, she will instantly get seriously ill.

Most people with obsessive-compulsive disorder are aware, at least on some level, that their obsessions and compulsions are excessive or unreasonable. Their behavior distresses them, takes up a lot of time each day, and seriously interferes with normal life. People with OCD have trouble functioning in everyday situations, at school, at work, and in relationships.

When someone with OCD is prevented from acting out the compulsive behavior, or tries to resist it, anxiety builds up to an amazing extent. The only way they can relieve the anxiety is to finally give in to the compulsive behavior. After a while, rather than constantly resisting and then giving in to the impulse, people end up trying to incorporate obsessive-compulsive behavior into their daily life. That works to an extent—if you get up early enough, you can check that you locked the front door many times and still get to work on schedule—but eventually the obsessive-compulsive behavior ends up replacing a lot of normal behavior.

## A Spectrum Disorder

OCD and eating disorders have a lot in common. For starters, both behaviors often start in adolescence or young adulthood. Both disorders involve persistent and intrusive thoughts; both involve a lot of ritualistic behavior; and both are spectrum disorders. In other words, the condition can range from very mild to very severe, across a spectrum. In its very mild form, OCD is extremely common. Almost all of us have some ritualized bit of behavior that we use, consciously or not, when we're feeling anxious.

I'm famous among my family and friends for worrying about being on time. To make sure I'm never late, I always set my clocks ten minutes ahead of the real time. Every night at bedtime I obsessively triple-check my alarm clock to be sure it's absolutely set for on, not off, and that it's absolutely set for AM, not PM I also triple-check the same things in the battery-powered backup alarm clock I set just in case the power goes off in the night—plus I triple-check to be sure the batteries in that clock are fresh and won't run out overnight. It's time-consuming, it's unnecessary, and it annoys the people around me, but if I don't do it, I get extremely anxious and feel convinced that I will oversleep the next morning and be late for everything—not only all that day but for the rest of my life.

I'm also famous for being very compulsive about the framed photographs on my office desk. They're arranged in small groups that have a particular meaning for me, and I get very upset if they get out of order or moved. I notice instantly if that has happened, and I can't be comfortable or concentrate on anything else until they're rearranged in exactly the right way.

Some of my friends are much the same. They're compulsive about organizing their time. They need to know exactly what their schedules will be every day for at least a full week in advance. They keep elaborate calendars with all sorts of color coding and tabs for different activities and appointments, along with detailed lists of everything they need to do each day. The good part about this is that they're never late and they never forget to do something that was planned. The bad part is that they have to spend a lot of time each day thinking about their schedule, updating, revising, and ultimately changing it, and coming up with new and improved systems for keeping track of all the details—even when planning a vacation. It's only when they have every hour of every day on their holidays blocked out well in advance and filled with an activity that they feel they can relax.

Many people incorporate at least some ritualized behavior into their everyday lives. Many musicians, actors, dancers, athletes, and other performers follow a special routine for their behavior before a performance, eating only particular foods, for instance, or doing a particular set of warm-up exercises in exactly the right order. Watch any professional baseball player coming up to bat and chances are you'll see a whole suite of ritualized behaviors.

Within reason, obsessive-compulsive behavior can actually be desirable as a way to channel anxiety and relieve stress. But when the behavior starts to interfere with daily life, or starts to cause distress to the individual, it turns into a disorder that needs treatment.

# Anxiety and Identity

Because many people with severe anxiety and perfectionism don't really have a well-developed identity of their own that could help them cope with the constant feeling of dread, they unconsciously turn to an eating disorder instead. The illness isn't a choice—it's usually more of an accidental discovery—but it works for them. An eating disorder may not be the ideal solution, but at least it's an identity of a sort, a way to keep the endless anxiety under control.

Being truthful and honest right from the start with my patients helps to break down their eating disorder traits. What I have learned is that I can't change their basic personality, nor can I keep them from experiencing anxiety. Instead, I can teach them how to live more effectively with their anxiety and how to navigate through change without taking refuge in the obsessive identity.

# FOUR

# Seeking Identity

*The individual* with an eating disorder sees herself as a performer on a stage, acting a role and seeking approval from the audience. Her performance is never over, however, and she never gets to remove her makeup, change out of her costume, or lead an independent life offstage. The person with an eating disorder is adept at picking up cues from the outside world. Unfortunately, that same person is not so good at listening to her own intuition or developing her own expectations. She has trouble creating an identity of her own, until she discovers that having an eating disorder is a great way to define herself.

Individuals with eating disorders *become* their disease, 24/7. Even among those who have had an eating disorder for only a short time, the illness preoccupies them completely, encompassing everything they do. They become cocooned within the disorder, and only something external can make them come out.

## Carol's Story

When Carol was seventeen and a star student in high school, she noticed that her mother was having trouble getting up in the morning, going to bed early, and constantly complaining of fatigue and headaches. Carol's parents were divorced, and her father was long gone from her life. Increasingly concerned about her mother, Carol took charge. She got her mother to finally see a doctor, who diagnosed her as having advanced cancer. Now Carol really had to take charge. As her mother's condition deteriorated, their roles reversed. Carol became the housekeeper, the cook, the nurse—the overall caregiver—while her mother became dependent, due to her illness. By never asking for help from anyone and managing to keep her grades up at school, Carol created a façade not just of normalcy, but of bravery and perfection. As she got caught up in her mother's needs and the increasing anxiety they brought, Carol began neglecting her own needs. Ironically, as she began to pay more and more attention to her mother's nutrition, Carol started skipping meals herself, and eating only restricted amounts when she did eat. By controlling her own eating, and by taking on a very strong identity as a caretaker, Carol was attempting to control her mounting anxiety.

Carol chose to attend a local college so she could be with her mother. Sadly, when Carol was a sophomore, her mother died. Carol now found herself with a strong identity as a perfectionist caretaker who also had an eating disorder—but she no longer had anyone to take care of. It took her mother's death for Carol to acknowledge her eating disorder and seek treatment for it. But even though she was seeing a therapist, she wasn't ready to drop her caregiver/eating disorder identity. In fact, she carried it forward to the next level. She chose to major in psychology and go on for an advanced degree so she could become a therapist herself. (This career decision is almost an automatic one for many young adults who have taken on the caretaker role, a role that is also often an aspect of the eating disorder identity.) Carol, not surprisingly, chose to work with people with eating disorders. This decision kept her not only in her comfort zone—now she was a professional caretaker—it also trapped her into an identity that prevented her own recovery. Because she disclosed to patients that she was a "recovered" anorexic, Carol gained credibility with her patients, and because she spent her days (and often evenings as well) surrounded by all the different aspects of eating disorders, she never fully let go of her eating disorder identity.

---

### *The caretaker role is often an aspect of the eating disorder identity.*

---

Carol thought she was an effective therapist because she had personal experience with an eating disorder. But because she was still within her own disorder, she identified too closely with her patients and couldn't maintain the objectivity that a professional needs. She started to feel more and more inadequate as her patients failed to improve or even relapsed. Eventually her sense of herself as a fraud, and the guilt and shame that came with that feeling, intensified to the point where Carol herself had a major relapse into severe anorexia.

As part of the therapy that helped her recover again, Carol was finally able to look rationally at her career choice. She realized that she had followed the path into becoming a therapist because it seemed a natural fit for her caretaker identity. She had thought she was in charge of making that decision, but she really wasn't. Her eating disorder identity was seeking ways to keep her within the framework of anorexia—and becoming an eating disorder therapist was the perfect tool for that.

As a teenager Carol had taken on the caretaker role out of necessity, at a time when she should have been exploring her own interests and developing relationships. Then in her work life as an adult, she became invested in an area that demanded a lot from her but gave her little grasp of the world beyond eating disorders. In our sessions, she and I talked a lot about the outside interests she had once had and where her passions truly lay. She came to realize that she enjoyed caretaking and wanted to continue helping people, but not as a therapist. She also came to realize that she didn't want eating disorders to be a controlling part of her life anymore, and that she needed to have interests in life outside her career. Carol was able to use her advanced degree and psychology credentials to move out of direct therapy and into a rewarding job as a program director for a healthcare company. Today, although she works long hours, she also knows when it's time to leave the office. Carol's anxiety and perfectionism are still with her, but she's learned to push them into the background noise of her life and not let them control her. Most of all, Carol has learned to open herself to the world around her and become a part of it.

# Who We Are, Who We Appear to Be

As children and adolescents—and even as adults—we all struggle to develop our own identities as individuals. As we pursue our interests and learn what really intrigues us, we also discover ourselves. Intense and sometimes short-lived passions are a normal part of growing up. They should be encouraged whenever possible as part of developing a strong identity.

Fundamentally, most of us have a sort of internal mechanism that, from an early age, informs us as to who we are. But the individual with an eating disorder doesn't seem to have that internal mechanism. Driven by picking up cues from the outside world, not by his inner intuition, he works to meet the expectations of others. While he will usually pick up on positive expectations—accomplishments, good behavior, prestige, good appearance, the things that get a lot of approval from the outside world—unconsciously he learns only how to perform so as to get the maximum amount of recognition. A juggler and a chameleon, he plays to

---

Most people with eating disorders pick up on the things that get a lot of approval from the outside world, rigidly channeling themselves into activities that look good, rather than those that feel good to them. They learn how to perform so as to get the maximum amount of recognition from others, rather than satisfy themselves. Seen from the outside, these people start out as great children and grow up to become competent adults. Their lives are highly successful, filled with accomplishment and praise. Inside, however, they feel a constant, anxious refrain: I'm not good enough.

the crowd, adopting interests that are most likely to bring him applause and approval instead of self-satisfaction.

Many of my patients appear to be happy achievers, but it's a façade. Internally, their psyche—which is just another way of saying their soul or personality—is actually quite fragile and unconsolidated. To put it another way, they simply don't know who they are. Because the façade of being perfect is all they have for an identity, they will protect it fiercely. The worst of it is that they're trapped. From a very early age, they've received so much positive reinforcement and external approval for the role they play that they can't afford to break out. What would happen to all that approval if they did? How would they deal with the hollowness inside? How would they cope with the inner voice that insists they're a fraud? Who would they be?

Individuals with eating disorders often feel as though they have no real identity of their own. Desperate to create one, they redefine themselves with an eating disorder, a performance that keeps them feeling in control. For many of my patients, that means that while they long for a successful career, good relationships with others, marriage, children, and being independent of their eating disorder, they are trapped in a cycle of self-doubt and an inability to set goals unrelated to the disorder. Their lives are on hold, with little accomplishment.

Another group of my patients, however, have become high achievers—and their eating disorder is just another "accomplishment." These are the CEOs, the supermoms who run complex households impeccably, the people who have attained the highest level of education or distinguished themselves in other ways. Likewise, their eating disorder has become a title of distinction, because they do it perfectly, maintaining and succeeding in their illness. But the pressure of anxiety continues to escalate, driving them onward toward more and more outward signs of success.

# The Fraud Concept

The person with an eating disorder feels like a fraud. He believes that no matter how well he's done in the past, no matter how many As or

---

*The fraud concept experienced by the individual with an eating disorder goes way beyond the self-doubt we all occasionally feel. It's an intensified sense of never being good enough, of being half a step away from disaster— from being found out.*

---

promotions he's achieved, no matter how many "I love you's" he's gotten from family or friends, he's just putting on an act. At the basis of this fraud concept is the belief that it's only a matter of time before he's found out. He's not really any good at all, and next time, he's going to fail and reveal what a fraud he really is. This isn't the occasional self-doubt we all feel. When the fraud concept is an integral part of your life, as it is for the person with an eating disorder, self-doubt becomes intensified. That horrible gnawing sense of not being good enough, of being just half a step away from disaster, is always there, no matter what.

The outside world may see these people as major achievers, but they see themselves as near failures. They downsize every genuine, hard-earned accomplishment, thinking to themselves that they just got lucky that time, that their luck is going to run out soon. To them, accomplishment only means more expectations to live up to. So, rather than enjoying their achievements, they see them only as an unavoidable step to even higher expectations and more responsibilities. That's why so many of my patients are driven overachievers. With more expectations and responsibilities, however, comes more anxiety and more dread of the future.

Something most of my patients have in common is their response to an anxious situation: It's totally disproportionate. The anxiety can become so severe that all of a sudden they can't concentrate or focus on future goals. Moreover, because the mind/body connection is very strong, disproportionate anxiety can create real illness. Headaches, nausea, stom-

*Very often the person with an eating disorder downsizes every genuine, hard-earned accomplishment, thinking to himself that he just got lucky that time. Unfortunately, a setback can be even more devastating, as the same person will believe that he's finally been found out for the fraud he really is.*

ach pain, diarrhea, back pain, and more are not uncommon when stressful situations arise. Sleep disturbances—a symptom of anxiety and also of the eating disorder—can leave the individual too exhausted to function in daily life.

I have a patient named Diana, an absolutely brilliant girl, who is an all-too-typical example of this. Diana had always had high anxiety levels and a strong tendency toward perfectionism. Combined with her high intelligence, these personality traits made her a very hardworking, straight-A student—until she turned sixteen. All it took was one B on one science test to totally demolish her. She completely lost any interest in school, dropped out, and got her GED only because her family pushed her to do it. The minute she dropped out of school, though, she had nothing to do and no identity. Her life now had a lot of empty time, and all of sudden, she wasn't in a situation where she could earn anyone's approval. She lost her identity as the perfect student and, for the first time in her life, felt the disapproval of her family and friends. Diana's sense of herself depended on being a good student, and now she wasn't a student at all. Isolated, without any other identity—and with no way to cope with a great deal of underlying anxiety—Diana was bewildered and desperate. Not surprisingly, she soon discovered that bingeing and purging her food intake gave her a sense of control in her out-of-control, anxiety-filled world. It brought the family spotlight back onto her, and it gave her a strong identity as a bulimic.

# Striving for Validation

It's easy to see how someone who strives for perfection but never feels she can attain it, someone who can see herself only as reflected in the approval of others, could come to have a distorted body image. Comparing her body to the perfect bodies shown in magazines and on TV, she believes that her body is less than perfect, even if her weight is normal. Less than perfect is something she has a very hard time accepting. The external approval she gets at that early stage just reinforces the goal of the perfect body. After all, eating healthier (as she rationalizes it) and exercising more are good things, right? The images of emaciated supermodels and actors she sees in the media reinforce the weight loss and exercise even more. She thinks, "If they can do it, so can I—and besides, they must be healthy if they're on the runways and in the movies." What is not recognized is that these professionals are paid a significant amount to have the bodies that they market to us as the norm.

As she loses more weight and exercises even more and starts to appear like the images that are marketed, she discovers something that finally goes beyond external approval: She attains not just an amazing sense of control but also a sense of identity that's not dependent on external validation. In the eating disorder she's finally found something she really can do perfectly and better than anyone else. She's also finally found something that gives her a real identity and fills her internal void. She now defines herself as a four-star eating disorder identity.

---

*"Less than perfect" is something the person with an eating disorder has a very hard time accepting.*

---

# Supporting the Disorder

Perfectionist tendencies, a preoccupation with food and weight, and a belief in a destination that can never be reached comprise the vicious cycle of the eating disorder.

Supporting an eating disorder can become a total preoccupation, if not a full-time job. Limiting and isolating, the eating disorder becomes a destination in itself, not a path to something better. For an individual with an eating disorder, isolation may be a way to stay protected and avoid moving beyond the eating disorder. In fact, she may see it as desirable, because it lets her focus more on the disorder, without any distractions.

## Marie's Story

I had a new patient recently who was more than a little reluctant to see me at first. When the time for Marie's appointment came, I went down the stairs from my office to my waiting area to meet her. Nobody was there, but there was a purse and a newspaper on the couch, the door was open, and I could hear screaming coming from the parking area. I went out to investigate, and sure enough, there was a sixteen-year-old girl who had locked herself in the car; her mother was pounding on the window, and the two were screaming at each other. Marie was no dummy. Her mother had lied to her to get her to my office, but once she was there, she saw the pictures on the wall of me at professional events and the eating disorder literature that was displayed and quickly realized she had been brought to see an eating disorder specialist. She wasn't interested— and she was really furious with her mother for tricking her.

I asked Marie's mother to please stop screaming and go back inside. Then I asked Marie to please crack the window so I wouldn't have to shout. She opened the window about half an inch. I told her, "I bet it wasn't your idea to come here today, and I bet your mother tricked you into it, but please come in and talk to me. I promise not to make threats or hold anything over your head. If you don't like me, that's Okay—just say bye and we're done."

She thought it over for a little bit and then came out of the car. When we walked into the waiting area together, I thought her astonished mother would have a heart attack. In our first session, I needed to align myself immediately with Marie and gain some form of trust with her. It worked. She has since returned for more sessions, and I feel we're making a lot of progress. What do we talk about? Anything and everything, but without significant emphasis on her eating disorder symptoms. We discuss what's going on with her schoolwork, what books she's reading, what movies she's seen, what she does with her friends, what her goals for the future might be. What I'm trying to help her discover is what truly interests her first—not what she thinks other people want her to be interested in. By talking about the things that interest her, Marie discovers her own passions. Some are new interests that she is pursuing on her own; others are old interests she put aside when people disapproved. What's important is that she's moving out of the narrow confines of her eating disorder and no longer defines herself by it. As that happens, the eating disorder itself fades more and more into the background and loosens its grip on her identity.

# The Identity Script

As a way to find out more about their self-identity, in our sessions together I ask my patients what they like to do and what their interests are. I often have a hard time getting the conversation started. It usually goes something like this:

DR. SACKER: What rocks your world?

PATIENT: What do you mean, rocks my world?

DR. SACKER: What are you interested in? What do you do with your open time?

PATIENT:        I don't have any open time—I'm too busy, I guess.
                When I have extra time I just sleep.
DR. SACKER:     Okay, but what do you do for fun?
PATIENT:        What's fun?
DR. SACKER:     Things that you enjoy, make you laugh, make you
                feel good about yourself.
PATIENT:        ?

If the conversation sounds wooden, that's because it is. The eating disorder identity leaves these individuals little room to express their true selves. They're caught in a space that has closed them off from any real pleasure or enjoyment in life and has narrowed their interests down to only one thing: their eating disorder. When they tell me they have no idea what fun is, they mean it. They won't allow themselves to relax and do something they enjoy just for its own sake; they don't see it as productive. Every action they take is considered in relation to the eating disorder. They're not interested in sports and don't play any, though they do work out. And when it comes to friends and family, I usually find that they have been gradually isolating themselves more and more. Their wider network of friends and family is now whittled down to a handful; they feel close to just a few people. Some will have long-distance friendships, have moved states away from their families, or create friendships online with no real social contact.

Often these patients think that rest and relaxation are a total waste of time. They don't think enjoyable things like good books, music, movies, and so on are really all that important. They see these things as negative and time-wasting. The whole concept of fun is negative to them, because it means they're not doing something productive. The truth is that these are some of the things that help form our identity. Our activities, our hobbies, our friends, what we read, what we listen to, and what we watch become part of our core. They also become effective ways to learn who we actually are and explore our potential and our talents. They expand our selves—exactly the opposite of what an eating disorder does. One of my patients once said to me, "You know, you ask me all these questions about

*Our activities, our hobbies, our friends, what we read, what
we listen to, and what we watch become part of our core.
They also become effective ways to learn who we actually
are and explore our potential and our talents. They
expand our selves—exactly the opposite of what an
eating disorder does.*

what I like, and I know I'm just making up the answers, because I don't
have any interests. The truth is that I don't really know what I like."

When I press patients who say they have no outside interests, I often
find that they're willing to talk about something that really does intrigue
them. They often preface it by saying, "This might seem weird, but. . . ." It
usually turns out that their interest isn't weird at all—it's just different from
the expectations of their friends and family. For perfectionists, wanting to
do something that doesn't meet the expectations of others is a real problem. They have trouble acknowledging that their own interests and desires
are different from what they think others expect of them and that they
don't always have to please others at the cost of their own needs or wants.

When patients don't appear to have any particular interests, we spend
time exploring the possibilities. I often have to point out that being
deeply interested in something doesn't mean you have to be perfect at
it—you're doing it just for the pleasure of it, not for the accomplishment
of it. I encourage my patients to explore art, music, writing, and other
ways of expressing themselves. To show my patients I practice what I advocate, I openly share my own passions for fishing, skiing, seeing movies,
traveling, and photography.

When patients do express a deep interest in something, I encourage
them to pursue it. Often, because perfectionists will quickly drop something they can't do to perfection, I'm encouraging them to return to an earlier interest. I've found that some of my patients once had deep interests
that other people deemed inappropriate. I had one idealistic patient who
was very interested in working with children. Her goal was to become an

elementary school teacher in an underprivileged neighborhood. Her lawyer mother and Wall Street father were very down on the idea, constantly asking her if there wasn't something else she wanted to do. What they were really saying was "You're an embarrassment to us—teaching isn't a serious profession. Do something that's more prestigious and pays more money." What individual can hold out against that sort of parental pressure? Her passion was smothered. Without realizing it, my patient picked the eating disorder instead. I was able to help her realize why she felt so torn between her desires and the pressure from her family, and I was able to help the family realize what their mixed messages were doing to their daughter.

# Losing the Eating Disorder Identity

Instead of moving ahead into positive possibilities, the person with an eating disorder gets stuck in them. He can't remember a time when he

---

An eating disorder can be a place of safety—something familiar and secure. The individual with an eating disorder will work hard to justify her decision to stay in the safety zone:

I find comfort in my disorder because I control it.

The eating disorder world lets me feel safe—it allows me to escape my fears.

I want the identity of the eating disorder.

What I fear most is that the outside world will take this away from me.

My destination is to remain in my eating disorder.

I have perfected this illness beyond measure.

My isolation isn't imprisonment, it's separation from my fears.

*If recovery is to take place, it's essential to learn how to push that eating disorder voice into the background.*

didn't have the illness, and he feels as if it's a life sentence. Moreover, he's got a lot invested in it. Having put a lot of effort into mastering that particular set of skills, he's going to be very reluctant to give them up after all that work. Given the choice between having extreme anxiety and panic attacks or having an eating disorder, he's going to go back to the identity he's used to—the identity of the disorder.

My patients often tell me they hear two inner voices, one telling them to give in to the eating disorder and the other telling them to struggle against it. The eating disorder voice is often the stronger. In fact, it's often as if the eating disorder voice is their best friend, because the voice brings them an irrational feeling of safety and trust. The eating disorder voice can come to sound very rational and normal.

When treating patients who have struggled with an eating disorder for a long time, I tell them this voice has nothing to do with their real, rational self. They always think I have no idea what I'm talking about, because the eating disorder voice is so strong and has been there for so long that it feels as if it is their only identity. Until they realize there is something more to their life than just their identity as a person with an eating disorder, that voice will remain strong.

But once they start to realize that it's perfectly normal to have multiple identities—that is, to have multiple roles to play, primarily as individuals, but also as family members, employees, friends, and so on—the eating disorder identity starts to recede into the background, overshadowed by healthier identities. When I help my patients discover their true identities and learn what their passions and interests are, they find that the eating disorder voice no longer has the same value to them. It's still there, and it may never totally disappear, but it no longer has any power over them. It becomes only the background noise of the rational mind.

*Eating disorders are so intense because, to the individual who has one, there's nothing to replace it. They don't want to stop. They put a lot of intensity into the disorder, and it becomes a safe place for them. They know their illness better than any other aspect of themselves, because they have become their illness.*

Because I think it's crucial to help patients learn how to push that eating disorder voice into the background, I encourage them to read books that have nothing to do with eating disorders. As I point out to my patients, they could write their own book about eating disorders, so why read one? Because many of my patients are perfectionists who are very goal-oriented and won't let themselves do something just for the fun of it, I often give them constructive "assignments," suggesting books and movies they might find engaging. I try to have them do things that take them away from their negative self-image and give them something to talk about besides themselves and their eating disorder.

## Shawn's Story

Years ago I treated a boy named Shawn who was very overweight. In the course of treatment, we talked a lot about how he needed to see beyond his physical appearance and that there were other things in life besides being slim. Shawn lost some weight while he was in treatment, but he stopped seeing me before he got down to a normal weight. Ten years later, Shawn made an appointment to see me again. I barely recognized the twenty-something man who walked into my office. He had grown into a tall, handsome, and very heavy man who clearly weighed over 300 pounds. Shawn had gone to a top-ranked university and earned an MBA. He was now a very successful financial analyst.

When I asked Shawn why he had decided to see me again, he said, "I think I'm ready now."

"Ready for what?" I asked.

"Ready to finally lose weight," he replied.

"And what makes you think you're ready for that?" I asked.

Shawn's answer really surprised me. He said, "Because I've decided that I really want to learn how to mountain bike."

I knew from our long-ago sessions that Shawn was a big sports fan even as a child. I was delighted that his passion had finally become something that he was willing to let into his life in a constructive way. I also knew from our long-ago sessions that Shawn was a very bright guy who always wanted an explanation for everything. I decided that if I was going to treat Shawn, he would have to do some preparation first. I told him, "Before we get started, I want you to go out and buy a good book on human metabolism and physiology. I want you to read it carefully and then call me to set up our first session."

Shawn did as I asked, buying not just one book on the subject but several, including the standard textbook used by medical students. When he arrived for his first appointment, he knew more than I did about nutrition and was ready to put all that knowledge into action. That meant we didn't have to spend a lot of time talking about dieting in our sessions. Instead, we could focus on how Shawn used food to soothe the intense anxiety he felt. Because he had been overweight since childhood, Shawn had felt he was destined to be overweight for the rest of his life. He couldn't see any other path for himself aside from the one he was on, with all the physical limitations obesity brings. His identity was as a fat person.

At the same time Shawn was having ongoing sessions with me, he hired a personal trainer to build muscle tone. He began training on an exercise bike. He was laughed at when he first arrived in the gym. Over the course of a year, he lost a significant amount of weight in a very healthy way. He began mountain biking in a beginners' league. He looked better, he felt better, he was more confident, and he was with a new group of mountain biker friends. Most important, the anxiety that he once smothered with food was under control. By increasing his exercise level so markedly with a sport he really loved, Shawn had found a different, much healthier way to calm himself and feel safe. He no longer felt the need to be protected by layers of fat. Through his mountain biking travels, Shawn began to meet people and participate in other activities. He became much less isolated.

Shawn's own words about his transformation are very revealing. He recently wrote to me, "When we began treatment I thought that weight and food controlled me and that I was sentenced to be overweight the rest of my life. I used being overweight as a way to justify all the problems and difficulties in my life. Whenever I would diet and lose some weight, someone would tell me how much better I looked. That would immediately make me go off the diet, because I knew that if I slimmed down I wouldn't be able to blame my problems on my weight. I wouldn't be the fat guy anymore. I'd have to be my own self, and I wasn't sure who that was. It was safer to just stay heavy. I've learned that the diet is the enemy."


For the patients who limit their activities, I teach them to learn from reading the words in books and hearing the dialogue in movies so they can create new interests and form new identities. Learning from other voices, both written and spoken, diminishes the power of the eating disorder voice. The patient learns that there's more than one kind of voice—and that those other voices have something valuable to say. Because patients can read books and watch movies in the comfort of their own home, they're not forced to face their socialization fears at the same time. They can focus on what they're reading or listening to in a safe place. Particularly for isolated patients, who often feel unsafe in the outside world, my "assignments" become a safe method for learning ways to create healthy identities within themselves.

OUTSIDERS:    Why do you want to stay like this? Don't you want to move out of the disorder and back into normal life?

PATIENT:    What other choices are there? I don't see anything better for me.

OUTSIDERS:   I don't understand why you won't change. You've been hospitalized so many times. Why go deeper into it?

PATIENT:   It's safer this way. I know you can't understand that.

OUTSIDERS:   What do you mean I can't understand? You're not even trying to get better.

PATIENT:   I don't have anything to say to you. Nothing can make this go away. I have tried, more than once, but I'm tired of trying.

OUTSIDERS:   Have you really tried? I don't see you changing anything. You never answer my questions—it makes me feel very frustrated.

PATIENT:   Well, join the club. I get frustrated with myself, too. I'm trying to answer your questions, but most of them don't even make sense to me.

OUTSIDERS:   You're just not hearing me. I keep trying to talk to you but you never listen.

PATIENT:   When I do respond, all you do is criticize my answers. It's safer and easier to just not answer at all.

OUTSIDERS:   Here we go again. You're just giving up.

PATIENT:   How is this giving up?

OUTSIDERS:   You won't stay with any conversation that's directed toward you.

PATIENT:   Fine. Let's talk about me. What do you want to know?

OUTSIDERS:   Why hasn't anything we've done for you helped?

PATIENT:   Define "help."

OUTSIDERS:   We've given you the best therapy and programs we can find, but I'm at a loss about where to go now.

PATIENT:   Nothing has helped because I wasn't ready.

OUTSIDERS:   What is it going to take for you to be ready?

PATIENT:   [Silence]

The dialogue comes to a dead end at this point. The person trying to help feels angry and frustrated. The person with the eating disorder feels completely misunderstood and frustrated—all the more reason to cling to the eating disorder identity they know so well. The outside world and the eating disorder world seem to be on parallel tracks—they can never meet.

# Where We Are, Where We Want to Be

We all set goals. We all have destinations, places in life where we want to be. Perhaps it's making the track team at age ten, or making partner at age thirty. Maybe it's becoming a husband or wife, or having a child. Or maybe that goal is a magic number on the scale or the size of clothing you want to wear. Whatever it is, our goals—and the process of reaching them—become part of who we are.

If your goal is to achieve the ultimate weight, you tell yourself that slimness is a good thing, that a smaller size of clothing is a desirable destination. And it can be. You're feeling better now that you're restricting your food intake and exercising more. You're losing weight and moving toward your goal. You have a point in the future on which to focus, not to mention a point on the scale. That keeps you busy. Ironically, you're both focused and distracted: focused on your weight and what you need to do to achieve that perfect number, distracted from the anxieties that would normally preoccupy you. If only you could nip and tuck your body through weight loss, you could be an absolutely perfect person.

As you continue to work toward your goal, as your destination becomes closer and perhaps harder to attain, you may deny yourself further. That doesn't seem such a bad thing in itself; every goal requires sacrifice. But when sacrifice itself becomes the goal, the end point keeps shifting

---

*The individual with an eating disorder denies herself and her own needs. She becomes a traveler without a destination, lost to the identity of an illness when one denies themselves and their own needs.*

---

and an eating disorder can take hold. You become like a traveler without a destination, lost to the identity of an illness.

That's what happens to the person with an eating disorder. Denying herself and her own needs, she imagines some future when a magic number is reached and everything will fall into place. Conversely, instead of working toward some perfect place or time, she may be restricting food (or bingeing or purging) to keep the feelings at bay. Rationally, she may know that she's fooling herself, but she can't let go of the idea—or of the ideal.

# The Illusion of Control

Individuals use eating disorders to pursue the illusion of control over their lives. It works like this:

**Anorexia:** Controlling through restriction

**Bulimia:** Controlling through bingeing/purging or overexercising

**Binge eating disorder:** Controlling through periods of extreme overindulging

**Compulsive overeating:** Controlling by filling emotional voids with food

The irrational mind makes these people believe that their eating disorder is putting them in control, but from a rational standpoint this is clearly an illusion. No matter where they are on the spectrum of eating disorders, the eating disorder is in control of them.

Breaking this illusion of control is at the core of effective therapy. When working with my patients, I help them find their passions and use them as a way to reinforce their new healthy identity. The rational mind becomes more capable of seeing just how irrational the eating disorder identity is. And as the eating disorder identity loses control, the irrational thinking and behavior that are central to it start to diminish. The more they diminish, the more the rational mind can reassert itself and diminish them further. What allows this to happen is that the space the eating disorder once filled is now filled by a deep passion. This passion fills the void that is left when the eating disorder subsides, and the eating disorder identity is replaced by a healthier, rational identity.

Our true identity comes from within. Discovering the things we love to do, the things that give variety and interest to our lives, is central to forming our own identities. When people with eating disorders discover their passions, they discover their own true selves, and the eating disorder self starts to lose its control over them.

# FIVE

# Breaking Free

*It's almost impossible* to treat someone with an eating disorder unless that person really wants to get well. That sounds straightforward enough, but part of having an eating disorder is strenuously denying that you do. I've had patients who were hospitalized and close to death tell me that they felt just fine and were ready to go home now. People have walked into my office with stick-thin arms and legs and told me they were too fat. Some come and tell me that their anorexia, bulimia, binge eating, or compulsive overeating isn't a major health risk, it's a lifestyle choice and that I have no right to interfere in it. Other patients arrive knowing they have a serious problem and are desperate for help, but unable or unwilling to make the changes that will really make a difference.

## Therapy Begins

Treating someone with an eating disorder actually begins prior to the patient being seen: She decides to seek help. Okay, sometimes that decision is forced on the patient by a concerned parent, spouse, friend, or doctor, but for the most part, patients walk through my door willingly. The real question is whether they truly want to get better, because without a hint of that desire, therapy goes nowhere. Often they don't really intend to change. They're coming just as a way to get concerned people to leave them alone.

It's my job to evaluate patients' desire to get better, and I'm pretty direct about it. I tell them that if they want to get better, I am there for them. If they don't, I can offer a compromise. I'll either wait until their motivation changes, or refer them to another therapist. My direct approach often pays off by making the patient think hard, perhaps for the first time, about whether she really wants to be in my office or not. More often than not, these patients decide that they do want to come back, and we can start making some progress.

# Fran's Story

Consider Fran. Twenty-three when we first spoke, Fran told me on the phone that she had been suffering from bulimia for thirteen years. In that time she had sought treatment from eight different doctors and therapists, yet she felt that her condition had become worse than ever. It's hard to tell from just a short telephone conversation if someone really wants help, but something in Fran's voice told me I might be her last chance. She agreed to see me at my office a week later.

Fran arrived at my office right on time and by herself. That immediately told me two things. First, being on time is usually a positive sign. Someone who's not sure about whether she wants treatment or not will often cancel or reschedule that first appointment. Many of my patients cancel and reschedule their visits several times before finally coming to the office. Others cancel their first appointment or just don't come. When I call to follow up, they may tell me the problem has been resolved or they've decided to work with someone else. Sometimes they just hang up on me—and sometimes they call back again months or even years later.

Secondly, because Fran arrived by herself, I knew that she was most likely seeking my help on her own. No family member was pressuring her into it or was escorting her to make sure she got to the office. That could be a positive sign of someone ready to take charge of her life.

When I first met Fran, she appeared to be a normal weight for her height, as are many people with bulimia. Her feminine contours were hidden under layers of clothing. She wore a baggy sweatshirt over an extra-large shirt, with a T-shirt underneath. Her jeans were baggy, too. She wasn't wearing any makeup, so I could easily see the dark rings under her eyes. Her long hair was parted in the middle and clearly hadn't been styled or trimmed. The overall impression I had of Fran's physical appearance was of someone trying to hide herself.

Fran and I quickly settled down to talk. I wanted to see past her label of bulimia and get to know her as a person. At the same time, I wanted her to see me not as just another therapist but as someone who was really interested in her, not just as another case of bulimia. That first session is where the connection is made.

From the outset, there were three vital things I needed to know from Fran:

1. How serious was she about wanting treatment?
2. How serious was she about wanting to stop the eating disorder behaviors?
3. Was she an immediate threat to herself or others?

During that first interview, I tried to get some clues that would answer those crucial questions.

I asked her to tell me, in her own words, a bit about herself and her family background. She told me that her father was an alcoholic and that while her parents were still married, their relationship was extremely combative and had been for years. She was the oldest of three children. Despite the stresses of her family life, Fran had been a good student in high school and had graduated from a prestigious liberal arts college. Once she lost her identity as a student and had to face the real world, Fran had trouble finding a direction in life. Because she was clearly intelligent and well educated and did well at interviews, Fran was able to

---

*I ask only two things of my patients: ultimate trust and a willingness to change.*

---

talk her way into a number of jobs. Her bulimic behavior kicked in at night, however, and left her feeling exhausted, bloated, and guilt-ridden in the mornings. She would then often be late for work or not show up at all, and would be fired within a few months. By the time she came to see me, Fran felt overwhelmed by her illness. She knew she needed to break out of the cycle of bulimic behavior, but she didn't know how.

Fran and I then talked about her eating disorder. She said her bulimia had begun while she was in middle school and never really stopped, though there had been periods when it was less severe. When I asked her to rate how severe the problem was right now, she said, "If I really want to be honest, I am worse now than ever before. My parents are threatening to throw me out of the house." It's not easy to live with someone with bulimia, especially if the binge/purge behavior is occurring frequently. At that point the person is often very secretive and touchy and incapable of participating in family life. Not only was Fran rapidly driving away her family support system, her bulimic behavior at night had made her almost unemployable. She was in serious danger of losing both her home and her job.

Fran went on to tell me about her previous attempts to stop the behavior. "I've seen eight different therapists and nutritionists," she told me, "but all they ever wanted to do was weigh me and talk about what I ate and what I vomited. I tried going to an eating disorder support group, but that didn't help me much at all. The other people were more messed up than me." She continued, telling me that one therapist had prescribed an antidepressant, and that it had helped somewhat. But, she said, "The only times I ever felt I was getting any better were when we didn't keep talking about my screwed-up family or how much I weighed or how often I threw up."

"Okay," I said, "let's just push past the eating disorder stuff and talk about you instead. Give me three words that tell me how you're feeling at this moment." Fran's words were telling: "I feel anxious, overwhelmed, scared."

Her response wasn't all that unusual, considering the decision to seek treatment is never an easy one—and anxiety is a major underlying issue for almost all my patients. As for feeling overwhelmed and scared, that's not unusual either. The prospect of giving up an eating disorder is overwhelming and scary. Bulimia creates a sort of numbed state that at first seems to decrease the anxiety. What brings the anxiety back is when you get pushed to deal with the bulimia, to acknowledge it or move out of it. To be willing to face the anxiety by starting therapy is a big step.

The more I talked with Fran, the more I felt that there was a smart, funny person underneath her bulimia—and that the last person to realize that was Fran herself. As our session went on, I felt that Fran had given me positive answers to the first two important questions: She was serious about seeking treatment and she really wanted to get better. The answer to the third question also became clear to me. Fran's bulimia was so out of control that it could start to pose a serious threat to her life. Her family and work situation were rapidly spinning out of control as well. I felt that a higher level of care, such as a residential treatment program, would be very helpful for Fran. I also knew that it would take at least several more sessions before Fran would trust me enough to give that idea serious consideration.

Finally, I asked Fran to tell me how she saw herself. Who was she, really? She answered, "I have bulimia."

"Yes," I replied, "you have bulimia, but that's not who you *are*. Who's the person that happens to have bulimia?"

She didn't have an answer.

# High Expectations

Individuals with eating disorders have very high expectations of themselves. Moreover, they believe that others have equally high expectations of them, even if that isn't really true. Constantly holding yourself

*An eating disorder can feel like a personal refuge, a safe place where there aren't any expectations.*

to such an impossibly high standard, constantly feeling that you're failing, can create a huge amount of anxiety. The eating disorder can become a personal refuge from that anxiety, a safe place where there aren't any expectations. If you come out of that safe place, the overwhelming expectations will start all over again. "If I get better, I'll have to go back to being a perfect person," says the eating disorder mind-set. "I'd rather stay sick." For many patients, the concept of better equals "I'm fat." What they really mean by fat is imperfect and out of control—the things they fear will happen to them if they let go of their eating disorder identity.

## What Does Wellness Mean?

If you have an eating disorder and start to get better, eventually you reach the magical weight—whether by gaining or losing—whereby nobody is going to see you as sick or having an eating disorder anymore. But to the person with the eating disorder, wellness doesn't just mean gaining or losing, or looking and feeling better. It means that nobody is going to take care of you, that the attention you got because of the illness will go away, that you're not going to have the eating disorder identity anymore. It means that you're expected to return to the real world. Wellness means you have to ask yourself, "Now what?" That's a terrifying question that the person with an eating disorder may not be ready to answer. It's much easier to just not ask it by staying in the identity of the eating disorder.

Individuals with eating disorders stay in an internal conflict with food by eating in a ritualized pattern every day—they know exactly when and what they're going to eat. The ritual takes away all their other feelings and makes them feel as if they're in control. Attempting to treat someone who's in this space is almost impossible. In fact, it can be counterproductive, because the patient will simply tighten her grip on the illness. In addition, if external resources such as hospital programs are brought up prematurely, the bonds of trust and honesty between a therapist and a patient can be destroyed.

# Focus on Recovery

One of the things I teach my patients right from the start is that they need to reduce the internal and external expectations attached to getting healthy. The focus needs to be on getting well. And even after they get better, they still don't have to do anything they don't feel ready for. For a typical patient, the expectations come both from within, driven by her own perfectionism, and from without, driven by our weight-obsessed society and the demands of family and community. By reassuring the patient that all she has to do is get better, I help her learn to manage her anxiety and get away from her perfectionism. At the same time, our discussions move further and further away from food and eating issues and more into exploring other aspects of her inner self. As we do, other interests begin to compete with the eating disorder and displace it from the forefront. Once a patient can start getting away from the obsessive thinking that characterizes an eating disorder, we're starting to make some real progress.

It's important for families to understand this part of the process and not put pressure on the patient. Statements like "Look what you're doing to your family," or "This is destroying your mother," or "We took a second mortgage on the house to pay for your treatment," or "We'll do anything to help you get better" only make the situation worse. They increase the shame and guilt the patient already feels, and they make the patient feel that she has to live up to more expectations. The therapist should do what

*Introducing positive interests to compete with the eating disorder can displace it from the forefront. And once a patient can move away from the obsessive thinking that characterizes an eating disorder, progress can be made.*

he can to move the focus away from the family and away from things that make the family feel responsible or guilty.

It's important, also, for loved ones to drop the negative attention that often comes with an eating disorder. Fran's case is a good example of how negative attention from the family can play a major role. Her parents had a very combative relationship; she had two younger siblings. Although outwardly the family appeared happy, the situation at home was very tense. Fran felt that she had to protect her mother and siblings from the community disapproval that would happen if the true family situation ever became known. Her way of doing that was to become the problem child, the one with the eating disorder. That kept the attention focused on her, not because she wanted it, but because it deflected attention from her mother and siblings. Fran used her illness to hide her family's dysfunction. Obviously, Fran didn't deliberately choose to have an eating disorder, or consciously decide that bulimia was the best way to protect her family, but when she discovered as a young teen that bingeing-and-purging behavior helped her deal with her overwhelming anxiety, she also stumbled across something that worked within the context of her family situation. It kept the spotlight off the rest of the family, and it brought her parents together—at least a little.

Often parents and other family members are at odds over how to deal with the "sick" person. For the patient, this can pay off, because sometimes any attention is better than none. A very common situation, one I see played out often by the families of my patients, is one in which one parent thinks a child has a serious eating disorder that needs professional help and the other thinks that the child is just "going through a phase."

The parents squabble about treatment and the child gets a lot of both negative and positive attention. The more the parents fight, the more established and rewarding the eating disorder behavior becomes for the child. The child is now at the center of family attention and has a measure of control over the parents. It's often only when the physical signs of the eating disorder become unmistakable that the opposing parent finally has to admit that help is needed.

When the attention is positive, I ask the family to keep it going, especially when the patient is improving. This might seem like a time when positive attention wouldn't be needed as much, but in fact it's the opposite. The road to recovery is very slippery, and patients need all the support they can find along the way.

## Carla's Story

I had a patient several years ago who exemplified the whole problem of losing weight being equated with rising expectations. Carla was an only child in a deeply religious ethnic family. Her parents were very protective of her and sent her to a religious school. At the age of twenty, Carla knew very little about the real world. Because her mother took care of all the domestic household duties and so on, Carla also didn't know much about how to run a household.

Soon after she turned twenty-one, Carla got married to another member of her religious community. Suddenly, this very naïve and protected young woman was expected to be a wife, with the intimacy that was involved, and likewise run her own household. Her family, her new husband, and her community expected her to take on a new identity as a wife and, soon after, as a mother.

Carla tried hard to accomplish what her community expected, but she just couldn't cope with her new identity. She had never developed a strong identity of her own before her marriage. Afterward, she wasn't prepared to take on the major transitions that faced her: leaving her parental home, new household responsibilities, intimacy with her husband, and the prospect of becoming a mother. All those expectations were too much for her, and she began to binge and eventually became severely overweight. By the time Carla became my patient, she had spent several years in and out of residential and intensive outpatient eating disorder programs. She would appear to get better, but as soon as her weight went down, the expectations placed upon her went up, and she would crash again. The one person who could sometimes get her to eat a normal meal was her mother, but only if she ate at her parents' house. Her condition was causing a huge amount of family discord—her parents and her husband were fighting with Carla and with one another over what to do about the problem.

When I first saw Carla, she appeared to be very depressed—she kept her head down and didn't make eye contact with anyone. Her description of what was going on with her illness and how it was affecting her parents and her husband made me realize that I had to bring them into the therapeutic picture quickly. After a few individual sessions with Carla, we had a family session with her parents and husband. I started by telling them what a great job they were doing. Then I gently suggested that maybe it would be best if they backed off on the food issues and stopped the talk about having children. I wanted them to help Carla focus on other things. For instance, Carla had no idea how to do laundry. I asked her mother to teach her the basics, without ever bringing up eating and food while she was doing it. Pretty soon, Carla mastered all her household tasks. Her husband was delighted—and went from being someone who was very negative about her condition to someone who was giving her the positive reinforcement she needed. More important, his praise helped Carla transition from being a daughter to being a wife.

As Carla mastered other basic household skills, she slowly began to gain confidence and stabilize her weight. I still needed to meet regularly with the family to encourage positive reinforcement, but Carla was definitely making progress. The key here was not to create expectations too quickly, but for Carla to tell me what she was ready for.

Recovery for Carla was a slow process of gradual transition. The expectations that had once seemed so overwhelming started to become manageable as her skills and self-confidence grew. At the same time, her parents and husband changed how they reacted to her. They stopped being so critical and angry and tried hard to be positive and supportive. This made a big difference for Carla, because it reinforced the wellness rather than the eating disorder.

# Blame and Support

It can be easy to blame the parents, spouse, or nonsupportive community for being a part of an eating disorder. But in the end, what does it matter? Blame is counterproductive and only justifies the illness. The bottom line is you have a human being who isn't functioning well. It's my job to help that person figure out how to get better, and to do it I need the help of that person's whole community.

In the past, we worked backward. When we met with the family of a patient, we told them how they had a part to play in the illness picture. We told the parents what *not* to talk about—basically, we told them to tiptoe on eggshells around the patient and to avoid most sensitive topics. We made the parents feel guilty and defensive, and it didn't work.

What works better is involving the patient's community in the treatment, but in a positive way. Sometimes part of that positive approach is to exclude people. That doesn't mean rejecting them, but it can mean setting some boundaries. This needs to be done in a supportive way. If a mother, for instance, were told that she needs to stay away from her daughter because when they're together the daughter becomes completely dependent, the mother would almost certainly become very defensive and the therapy would get nowhere. If instead the mother is told, "You've been doing a great job here. Now there are a couple more steps you can take to help your daughter, but they're going to take some strategizing on your part. Take a step back and let your daughter do certain things for herself. You have to keep telling her you know she can do them and reinforce her when she accomplishes them." What this does is create a boundary and give the daughter her own space, but by having the

---

*Blame is a way to justify our own limitations.*

---

mother think she's doing it. In the end, the family needs to feel they had a positive role in the recovery, even if their part was to take a step back.

Just as I don't want the families to feel blame, I don't want patients to feel blame either. Blame is a way to justify our own limitations. Patients may say, "It's not my fault," but even so, most have an underlying belief that they *are* to blame.

Patients need to recognize that blame is connected to past scripts. As long as they stay in the past they cannot move forward.

To move beyond the concept of blame there needs to be consistent and concrete support for the patient, as well as the family.

# Changing Visual Perspectives

To the outside observer, someone with a serious eating disorder is viewed as either one end of the spectrum (too thin) or the other end of the spectrum (too fat). Individuals with eating disorders, however, have difficulty seeing themselves as they actually appear. Helping patients to see themselves as they really look is part of the rational aspect of changing the patient's perspective. I use a combination of digital photography and video as a way for the patient to begin to recognize an identity past her own eating disorder identity. Recording how the patients actually appear lets them see themselves from a different perspective, not just in their mind's eye. I ask patients to take pictures of themselves or to make a video that shows them walking and standing still, with front, side, and rear shots. Through discussion of the imagery of specific areas, such as the arms, legs, stomach, and central areas, the individual begins to create a dialogue of body dissatisfaction as well as a new reality of their true appearance. I also ask the patients to pick out three or four photos or video

*Individuals with eating disorders, however, have difficulty seeing themselves as they actually appear. Helping patients to see themselves as they really look is part of the rational aspect of changing the patient's perspective.*

scenes and ask them to explain, in their own words, how this tool was effective and how to apply their new perspective toward their wellness. It's a very valuable technique. Seeing themselves so objectively in only two dimensions leads to many "aha" moments.

Those insights can be scary but groundbreaking in shattering their illusions. When they realize that what they see in that eating disorder mirror isn't accurate, it helps them transition to a different space. It also builds trust between us, because they realize that what I've been telling them about their weight is true. I help them break the circus mirror and see themselves undistorted by their eating disorder.

On a practical and rational level, I ask my patients to give away their clothing when it no longer fits because they've gained or lost weight. Some patients with eating disorders will lose so much weight that they can fit into much smaller sizes, even children's clothes. They'll then start to gain a little weight, but when they feel their skin is starting to touch their clothes, they'll start to restrict again. To break this cycle I ask patients to donate the small sizes and wear clothing that's appropriate for their weight. When my heavy patients lose weight, I encourage them to get rid of their "fat clothes" and buy new clothing in an appropriate size. Some of them don't want to do that until they've lost some specific amount of weight, which means that in the meantime they're going around in clothing that looks oversized. When your clothes are baggy and don't fit, nobody can see that you are looking and feeling better. I encourage them to buy some nice new clothes while they're at an intermediate weight. The patients get the reward of shopping for fashionable new clothing that fits their new figure. More important, the process helps them focus on the present and the progress they're now making in therapy and takes away the focus on some distant future.

# Family and Community

The mother of one of my patients comes to joint sessions with her son. She always wants to discuss how he isn't eating and is exercising way too much. She talks the talk and is really very good with him, but one look at her tells me she's not eating herself and that she's an exercise junkie. She's saying one thing and doing another—and her son knows it perfectly well. That sort of contradictory parental behavior is very confusing, though in this case, it's turned out to be a good thing. Too often, parents give children the impression that adulthood is easy. Then, when the children get older and encounter difficulties, they think, "I must be really screwed up, because my parents never have these problems." My patient has come to realize that his mother has her own struggles with eating, and that realization has helped him understand his own problems.

When I first began to treat patients with eating disorders, I didn't really focus much on the eating patterns of the parents. I saw the eating disorder as something that sort of popped up in the family. I soon realized that there was more to it than that. As their child started to recover, a surprising number of parents would reveal to me that they too had experienced some form of disordered eating or some addiction in their past. Recently, scientific research has started to show what I have suspected for a long time: There is a genetic component to eating disorders. Genes alone don't explain the explosion of eating disorders we have seen in the past few decades, but it's clear to me that they play a role.

*As we say in medicine, genes load the gun but environment pulls the trigger. We live in a society that's optimally designed to pull the trigger on eating disorders.*

I have been fortunate to treat a lot of patients with very supportive families. I've also had to treat patients who had virtually no support from their families. Some of my patients have been brought to me not by concerned family members but by friends, teachers, coaches, and others who could no longer stand by while the family neglected or refused to acknowledge the problem.

What's going on here? In almost every case, it's denial. Sometimes a parent truly doesn't see the eating disorder behavior because it is well masked by the struggling child. But when the weight loss or gain gets severe, or when the evidence of bulimia (vomit all over the bathroom) or overeating (empty food containers and refrigerator) is almost impossible to ignore, some still choose not to see it. The reasons are many. Sometimes it's because they don't want to admit that their parenting might be part of the problem. Sometimes it's because they don't want to admit that their child is anything less than perfect, although of course that perfectionism could well be at the root of the problem. Sometimes it's because admitting the problem will bring shame on the family, or will call attention to additional family issues. Sometimes it's because another family member is severely ill or has some other problem that demands most of the family's attention. And, sadly, sometimes it's because the family is indifferent or estranged or simply doesn't exist.

Reclaiming the self from the depths of an eating disorder is never easy, no matter how supportive the family and community are. The way forward isn't always easy to see, and there can be many detours and potholes on the road. Recovery is a slow and uneven process, especially when, as often happens, it uncovers additional issues.

SIX

# PIRT: A New Approach

*I never realized* I had a systematic way of treating my eating disorder patients until I started reviewing my thirty-five-plus years in the field. In the process of preparing for a speech at a national eating disorder conference, I started to create an outline of my treatment approach. I wanted to focus on specifics, not generalities, and this forced me to really think through exactly what it was that worked—and didn't work—in my treatment methods. I was more than a little surprised to realize that the approach I had always considered very intuitive and free-form actually had a strong but flexible underlying structure. After I got over my initial reaction, my medical training kicked in. I realized that if my approach was systematic, that meant other people could learn how to use it as well.

## Four Fundamentals

I didn't plan to give my approach a catchy acronym, but PIRT turns out to be a pretty good shorthand way of referring to the four basic concepts of my treatment approach: Personal Interactive Rational Therapy. PIRT doesn't refer to stages of recovery, but to an approach that moves individuals

105

---

*Personal Interactive Rational Therapy: PIRT doesn't refer
to stages of recovery, but to an approach that moves
individuals toward recovery.*

---

toward recovery. Most important, PIRT helps with transitions, always the most difficult part of recovery.

It's one thing to be in the supportive, isolated environment of a treatment program for eating disorders. It's another thing completely to arrive back home from the program and have to cope with the world again, without the benefit of the insight and support a program can provide. Not surprisingly, many eating disorder patients have a hard time with change and transition. The anxiety they feel is so strong that they immediately fall back on the one thing they know they can rely on and the one place where they feel safe—their eating disorder. By using the basic concepts of PIRT, I've found that my patients can move away from their eating disorder world and learn how to navigate in the real world.

# Personal

My treatment approach with all my patients has always begun with the personal. I'm not a big fan of old-style impersonal medicine. I see the doctor/patient relationship as a partnership for positive change, which is why the personal aspect starts with the very first contact with the patient and continues throughout. For our work to be successful, I need to feel a personal rapport with the patient and with the patient's family. They have to feel comfortable with me as a person, not just satisfied with my credentials. They're feeling a lot of mixed emotions at that point—they're frightened, concerned, exasperated, and even angry—so, from the very start, I try to establish a nonjudgmental relationship where everyone feels

*Trust and the willingness to change are essential if recovery is to take place.*

he or she can be completely honest, without feeling defensive or as if he or she is being blamed for the situation. I'm very direct right from the start about the need for honesty, and I only ask two things from my patients and their families: trust and the willingness to change.

It's very important for the patient and the family to realize early on that I understand eating disorders as a medical doctor as well as an eating disorder specialist. I will quickly see through all the excuses, rationalizations, and avoidances they offer. I also let my patients know right up front that this isn't a game centered on food and weight. For example, right from the start I tell them that they know more than I do about nutrition—after all, most of them have been counting fat grams and calories for years. Almost always, they say, "How do you know that?" I just ask them, "How many calories in a bagel?" When they respond, "Small, medium, or large?" they see my point. When we discuss their weight, I point out that I know all the tricks and games they can play to try to fool me about weight loss and weight gain, and I won't fall for them. If they try to play the weight game, they're only cheating themselves and may not be ready for change.

I tell my patients that they can lie to me if they want—but that will only break down the entire relationship of trust we're trying to establish. I don't care what they tell me, as long as it's truthful. I've had patients scream at me and call me every terrible name in the world. It's not easy to take, but I'd rather be called bad names honestly than have a patient say nice things that are a lie. I tell my patients and their families, "Whatever you're going to tell me, it's got to be truthful. You have to tell me exactly what's going on and I have to believe you. If I find I can't do that, then we don't have a therapeutic relationship. And if that happens, then there's no reason for you to see me, because treatment won't be effective."

---

*Patient and therapist need to work as partners, not adversaries.*

---

In most cases, my patients are actually very relieved to hear me insist so strongly on honesty. Some will try to test me by telling me things they know I will immediately recognize as lies, but most stay honest because they know I'll see right through them. We quickly get past all the possible manipulations. I want my patients as partners, not adversaries.

During our first session I let my patients know that we're forming a mutual therapeutic relationship. How do we get there? Through mutual acceptance, explanatory discussions, open conversations, and identity assessments. We can usually establish a rapport quickly. Only rarely is a patient so angry or resistant that I can't break through, at least a little bit. I'm looking for the real person in there, the one I know is hiding behind the eating disorder. I want to get to know that person, to see things from her perspective, because that's the person who will form a therapeutic partnership with me.

## Dismantling Negative Patterns

A common theme for almost all my patients is the phrase "I'm never good enough." They'll tell me, "I'm a failure, I'm fat, I'm unattractive." What they don't tell me is "I get good grades," or "My boss thinks I'm the best worker he's ever had," or "I'm a really good teacher," or "My children respect me," or "My spouse loves me." They become fixated on the negatives and on what they perceive as failures and simply can't accept or see that they have any positive characteristics or achievements.

One of my patients, a forty-three-year-old named David, was a successful sales executive. He would give excellent, well-prepared presentations to clients and then take questions. If he felt he had messed up in the slightest way, or if he perceived a question or comment to be in the slightest bit critical, he would then beat himself up for hours afterward about it. Because he was a real perfectionist, what got lost in all that self-criticism was that his presentations usually went very well and he often made the sale. His obsessiveness and his perfectionism were major triggers for his eating disorder. Before presentations, he would binge and purge as a way to relieve the anxiety; afterward, he would do the same thing to relieve his anxiety over what he saw as a failure.

When he first described this pattern to me, he told me that at a recent presentation the client had asked him a question he couldn't answer. He didn't show it outwardly, but inwardly he was devastated by this "failure." I asked him, "How many positive things does it take to outweigh that one negative?"

"Nothing can outweigh that negative," he replied.

"Really?" I said. "What about the way you handled the question you couldn't answer? You told the client you didn't know and would find out, and afterward she told you how professional that was. And doesn't the fact that you got the sale count for anything?"

"Well, yeah, I did get the sale," he admitted. "Maybe I shouldn't worry so much about answering every question."

When a patient is a perfectionist with an eating disorder, the therapist can't just be a nodding bobblehead. He has to be personal and remind the patient of what he's accomplished, because he often can't recognize his accomplishments himself. The patient with an eating disorder has to be taught how to put things into perspective, how to consider the source when someone makes a comment that he interprets as critical. The therapist must help the patient work toward dismantling the irrational patterns. That means encouraging the patient to acknowledge his accomplishments,

---

*Very often individuals with eating disorders will become fixated on the negatives and on what they perceive as failures. They simply can't accept or see that they have any positive characteristics or achievements.*

---

remembering personal details about the patient, and being willing to bring up the positive achievements in a proactive way.

# Interactive

When I was in medical school, we were taught to be very remote and not reveal anything about ourselves to our patients. This was the old-style therapy, where the patient lay on the couch and the doctor sat beside it, unseen by the patient. How this was supposed to help anyone, much less a teenager with an eating disorder, was anybody's guess. My very first experience with this approach happened when I was a young resident just starting to work with troubled adolescents. I was told to do an initial evaluation of a fourteen-year-old young man named Robert who had come to the clinic for depression. I was also told my supervisor would be observing me through the one-way mirror in the interview room.

I did as I had been taught. I went into the room, introduced myself, and asked some open-ended questions that were completely neutral. I wasn't supposed to be directive or interactive in any way. So I asked all the right questions ("What brings you here today?" for instance) in the right detached, professional way, and nothing happened. Robert just sat there in absolute silence for forty-five minutes—he didn't say a single word. I went along and sat there in silence, too, but I was getting more anxious by the minute. Sweat was pouring down my back as I tried desperately to think of a way to reach this kid with my open-ended, non-interactive questions. At the end of the allotted forty-five minutes, I ended the session. Robert got up and walked out, still without saying a word.

When I walked into the evaluation meeting with my supervisor after the session, I was sure I had really blown it with this patient. To my astonishment, I was congratulated on how well I had handled the interview. I couldn't believe it—there had obviously been no communication between Robert and me, much less any therapy, yet my seniors were telling me it had been a good session.

A little to my surprise, Robert came back for his next session. This time, nobody was watching through the mirror. Rather than picking up using the same silent dialogue I had first used, I started off by telling him that our last session had caused me intense anxiety, and I assumed it had done the same for him. It was like flipping a switch. The look of relief on his face was amazing. He immediately told me that our session had made him extremely uncomfortable and that he had almost decided not to come back again. I told him we were in the same boat together, and with that common ground, we were able to start talking. He opened up, to the point where I had to slow him down. I didn't want him to disclose too much at once and then be afraid to return for additional sessions.

## The Problem with Labels

That was really the first time that I recognized the standard approach to therapy wasn't going to work for me. I couldn't stand those silences. What was effective was the interaction between two individuals, one of whom had training and background and really cared about the other one.

My therapy sessions are interactive and conversational. The most important part of the interactive aspect, however, is helping the patients explore themselves: their own thinking, reactions, and behavior. Most of all, we explore who the patient really is. The true identity—not the labels received from others. Many of my patients were labeled long ago by their families, schools, and communities. Some were told they were gifted, or perhaps stupid, others that they were fat or unattractive or would never be successful. Even being labeled as beautiful is something you might very much want to escape, if you didn't really feel all that beautiful when you had to cope with the real world. To escape from those labels, patients took on the eating disorder label instead—not by choice but out of a search for safety. It makes sense, in a way. A lot of them decided they'd rather be labeled as having an eating disorder than as a failure.

I spend a great deal of time with my patients exploring those labels. It can be a painful process, because sometimes the label has been applied unfairly. Patients can feel terribly betrayed when they realize that the labels that have been applied to them aren't really accurate. They often have high anxiety levels and obsessive-compulsive behaviors that can really get in the way of who they are, resulting in a misdiagnosis such as learning disabled or ADHD, and the label sticks.

All those labels and the visual illusions of the perfect body that are put out by our society, the media, family, and peers can lead to a negative distortion of the self. It's important that the patient be encouraged to see past that distortion and get to a point where she can communicate her own realistic wants and needs, not those that come from other people. That's why the therapy moves away from food, weight, and appearance to discover the patient's true passions and interests. When a patient can learn what really rocks her world, she can then find a way to use that rational thinking to help replace the eating disorder.

## Nora's Story

One of my patients, a woman named Nora, who was well into her thirties, told me that when she was six and in first grade, she had a crush on a boy in her class. He told her he really liked her, too, and asked her to meet him after school at the local park. When she got there, though, he was with some of his friends and they just laughed at her. He told her he didn't really like her at all and had just been fooling her.

I said, "You know, that's a major event in your life—it's not something to be embarrassed about. What happened after that?"

With those simple words of support, Nora was able to admit to someone other than herself how this one event had resonated throughout her life. It was at the core of all the difficulties she had experienced ever since with relationships. To help her see it in perspective, I used a personal anecdote from my own life. I told her about the time I was thirteen and went to a school dance. I was a pretty good dancer and I was dancing with this cute girl. Afterward she said to me, "It's kind of hot in here. Maybe we should go outside and cool off." Clueless adolescent that I was, I said, "It feels fine to me." She gave me a look that told me I was a total loser and walked away. When the next song came on, she was dancing with someone else.

Nora totally cracked up when I told her this story. She said, "You couldn't have been that dumb."

"Yep," I replied. "I was." What the personal story told Nora, without minimizing what she felt, was that her experience was really a universal experience. She's not the only person to have ever experienced rejection and humiliation, to have been naïve. Even her therapist has had his fair share of similar experiences.

# Rational

People with eating disorders are often hypersensitive to feedback or constructive criticism, even when they're not actually being criticized. They'll interpret a casual remark, often one meant in a friendly or supportive way, as a personal criticism instead. When someone with anorexia, for instance, hears a friend say, "You look so much better," or "You're looking good," she doesn't hear good things or a compliment. Instead, she hears "You've gotten fat" or, in her irrational mind, "You've failed!" She may immediately start restricting food again. An innocent remark can really devastate her. I help my patients learn to see these remarks as the positive statements they really are and to understand that other people also misinterpret things. I tell them, "You know what? Nobody likes criticism. Most of them just don't show it because they've developed a sort of outer shield. They can be a little more detached and not take everything quite so personally." That's where the rational aspect of therapy starts to come in, because my patients begin to understand the difference between what the irrational mind tells them ("I'm being criticized because I'm a failure") and what the rational mind tells them ("That was really a neutral remark or maybe even a compliment").

Being rational about food, eating, and body image isn't easy, but a rational approach is necessary to reinforce healthier, more positive thinking. The goal is to help the individual take another important step:

*As part of thinking rationally about their eating disorder, individuals need to learn how to redirect their energy into other channels—but healthier, productive channels, not just new manifestations of compulsive behavior.*

the move forward into an unknown transitional identity. This aspect of therapy helps patients look at rational concepts that will effectively redefine who they really are, and that can be a very scary thing. I can't sit there and take away someone's eating disorder identity until they have filled that void with something they see as more important to them.

Therapy can take a long time. For many patients, it takes months or years of therapy before they can even think of letting go of the eating disorder behavior and the identity that supports it. That transition can be a very difficult one, with false starts and sometimes even relapses. Patients who are compulsive overeaters, for instance, often lose a lot of weight during therapy. Now they need new clothes and can enjoy shopping for a new wardrobe—a fabulous reward for all that hard work. But for these patients, the transition to a slimmer self is difficult. When they look in the mirror, they find it hard to believe that their new reflection is really them. The reflection they see is still their former self. Rewarding their new behavior and the positive self-care it represents can often turn into a new compulsion. They channel the compulsive impulse into shopping. I've had patients who went on shopping binges and ran up thousands of dollars on credit cards in just one day. They continue to find satisfaction in outward appearances and not inward strength.

Obviously, this is a serious problem for both the patient and the therapist. As part of thinking rationally about their eating disorder, patients need to learn how to redirect their energy into other channels—but healthier, productive channels, not just new manifestations of compulsive behavior. When the old eating disorder behavior comes back under a new name, the patient must deal with it in a rational way to become aware of what the behavior is really saying. Often they have this idea that if they reach a certain weight their whole life is going to be different, thinking they're going to magically become a different person with a more positive identity. But the reality is that when they reach their new weight and fit into new clothes, they feel more anxious and shameful than they ever have before. They've never seen themselves as thin—they still feel fat. Now they're at a weight they've never been before and their anxiety levels are over the edge.

## Being Rational About Anxiety

Anxiety is the underlying issue here—not clothes or food and not even weight. I help patients understand on a rational level that no matter what happens in their lives, they're *always* going to feel anxiety. Learning how to live with it is a major core issue, one that the rational aspect of the PIRT approach can really help.

Before I can help my patients find ways to cope with anxiety, I usually first have to help them understand exactly what anxiety really is. Most of us know that anxiety is an internal sensation of uneasiness or dread in response to or in anticipation of a stressful situation, like an exam or performance review. When you're anxious, you feel nervous and edgy; your heartbeat may get faster, and you might break out in a sweat or need to use the bathroom. Generally speaking, when we're anxious, we know it. Not so with many of my patients. When they get that squishy, unpleasant, uncomfortable inner sensation, they don't recognize that it's anxiety. They don't know what it is—they often describe it to me as pain in their chest or stomach or as feeling sad. Whatever the feeling is for them, they don't like it, and they've learned that their eating disorder behavior relieves it.

In therapy sessions with my patients, we'll often be discussing deep issues and suddenly the conversation will veer off to food, weight, and appearance. At that point I'll say to the patient, "Whoa. Back up there. We were talking about you and now all of a sudden we're back to talking about how you look again. What are you feeling right now?"

The answer is usually something like "I'm feeling stressed" or "I'm

*When patients learn to recognize anxiety for what it is, they can begin to separate the feeling from the voice in their head that tells them to engage in eating disorder behavior. And only then can they finally stop associating anxiety with food.*

feeling nervous."

"That's anxiety," I tell them. "By focusing on your trauma, we raised some core issues, and that made you feel anxious. When you feel anxious, you feel that old familiar sensation in the pit of your stomach and you go right back to the old familiar groove of talking about your eating and your appearance. Whenever you feel anxious, your irrational mind is going to spin you right back into irrational thoughts about your body and your weight. But once you can recognize that what you're feeling is anxiety, you can block out the irrational thinking."

To help my patients learn to identify that anxious feeling, we sometimes do a little experiment. We sit silently together in my office. Pretty soon the patient's anxiety level begins to rise. After about ten minutes, I ask the patient how she's feeling. The answer is usually "Very anxious." When patients learn to recognize anxiety for what it is, they can begin to separate the feeling from the voice in their head that tells them to engage in eating disorder behavior. And only then can they finally stop associating anxiety with food.

The rational part is the next step. Now that you can recognize anxiety for what it is, what are you going to do about it? The answer is nothing. Individuals with eating disorders tend to be a lot more anxious than most people, but anxiety is part of being alive. I help my patients learn to see their anxiety in a rational light, accept it, and live their lives anyway. It's like waking up with a slight headache. It's not a great feeling, but you can manage to go on with your day and be productive anyway. And during the day, you might get so interested in something that for a while you forget you have a headache, even if it comes back later on when you're not as engaged. That's the approach I help my patients take with the anxiety they constantly feel. They learn that they don't have to process their anxiety all the time, because it's just going to be there no matter what. They learn to acknowledge it and then just push it into the background.

## Anxiety Masks the Identity

You can't create a new identity with just clothing or weight loss or outward appearance. Internally you're the same person, stuck with the same life issues. The problem is that when patients begin to recover, their family and friends think they feel as good as they look. They don't. In fact, this is a very fragile time for patients, because they still don't have any idea who they really are at this point. The high anxiety level this creates can often cause a relapse back into the safety of the eating disorder.

The patient begins to experience positive feedback that focuses on outward appearance. As the weight changes and the patient looks better, family members and friends start making appearance-based comments, like "You look so much better," or "You've gained weight." The comments seem supportive and helpful, and they're meant that way, but the patient doesn't always hear them that way. To the patient, the positive support can actually create anxiety, because she knows that while she may look better externally, internally she doesn't really feel a whole lot better. She's still searching for her identity, trying to figure out what she really looks like and who she really is.

This is a major transition point. When the patient reaches it, the therapist needs to provide guidance by using rational distinctions to block out the irrational eating disorder voice and triggering outside comments.

*A big part of recovery is learning to think about identity without automatically thinking about food or body image.*

At this point patients don't have a clue as to who they really are. They're probably experiencing a lot of anxiety and confusion. Now is when the therapist has to really walk them through the transition point, helping them to block out all the voices they're hearing from family members and friends. Everyone is responding in a positive way—which is good—but at this point everyone also assumes that the patient is "cured" and has become "normal." People figure it's time to stop talking about the eating disorder because, at least outwardly, it's been fixed. The patients don't see it that way. They know they're not "normal" yet, but they're also being told that they're no longer patients. The anxiety this creates can be overwhelming and is a leading cause of major relapse.

Other people think they're giving the right message and being supportive, but the reality is far different. What is the right message? One that doesn't focus on how great someone looks or how wonderful someone is, but a more low-key, nonjudgmental message that says you understand that she is going through a difficult and confusing time, and you're going to help her get back into the world. Simple statements like "I'm glad to see you" or "call me" are supportive and helpful. At this point a patient needs to be able to talk more about identity and a lot less about appearance and body image.

## Beginning the Transition

It's crucial to provide support as patients seek their true identity, but not to manipulate or pressure them with overwhelming expectations of "normalcy." I know that what they hear from their friends and family is going to be very confusing, so I give my patients a sort of prep course on how to find better ways to understand and communicate with family members and friends. For example, often when a patient returns home from hospitalization, the family wants to celebrate. Having a party in her honor at this confusing moment, however, is almost certain to do nothing but create intense anxiety for the patient. A smaller, quieter welcome

*Eating disorder patients are very sensitive to the people around them—they'll pick up on unexpressed emotions, unspoken disapproval, and false attitudes instantly.*

home—one that doesn't have food as a central element—makes the transition easier.

Sadly, many patients need to prepare for making the transition on their own. In many situations, the family just can't provide the right sort of support—too many changes have to be made by too many people in a very short period of time. Patients must grasp that they can't expect that the family has changed much or that friends are always going to say the right thing. Both sides need to know what to expect on a rational, realistic level. Eating disorder patients are very sensitive to the people around them—they'll pick up on unexpressed emotions, unspoken disapproval, and false attitudes instantly. They then become very suspicious and can end up in relapse when they realize the support they need isn't really there—that family members are trying hard, but their attempts to say the right things aren't working very well.

Therapists guide patients away from things that are unhealthy substitutes for their eating disorder and into areas that are truly important to them. Once they do find those new areas, they can process how that looks and how they can begin to reformat their life. I always know we're getting close to that point when a patient says to me, "How come we're not talking about food and dieting anymore?" Individuals with eating disorders would rather talk about food and dieting than anything else. As long as they can keep talking about food and weight and body image, they can stay away from what the underlying issues really are. When patients realize that they're no longer relying on their irrational thoughts, they're at the transitional moment where effective therapy begins.

# Therapy

Therapy and healing happen when patients choose to get well based on self-respect and trust. They actively choose to develop strong, protective identities as self-reliant individuals who have learned to accept their insecurities and anxieties and move on despite them.

It's not enough just to get to the root of whatever trauma has contributed to the eating disorder. Often there is no one specific event—the trauma is emotional and comes from not being heard, not being listened to, not being good enough, not getting any positive reinforcement. No matter what it is, if we get to it without having some sort of protective identity in place, the anxiety can become overwhelming. That can lead to a relapse—a retreat right back into the eating disorder.

Therapy isn't always easy to get under way. I've had a lot of very resistant patients. The honor of being the most resistant patient would belong to Hannah.

## Hannah's Story

I first met Hannah a few years ago, when she was sixteen and was brought, literally kicking and screaming, to my office. I was running a little behind schedule, so there was another new patient waiting to see me in the open hallway leading to my office. Hannah walked down that hallway calling her friend who brought her the vilest names at the top of her lungs, and knocking all my pictures off the walls on the way. I immediately brought her into my office just to stop the destruction. Without saying a word to me, she flung herself down on the couch, put her legs up on the coffee table, and began calling me horrible names at the top of her lungs. When she ran out of breath, she grabbed one of the pillows from the couch and threw it at me. At that point I said, "I have had many people in my life, and not one of them has ever articulated their anger as effectively as you have. Nothing personal, but there is no way I will see you under these conditions. That is the most disrespectful language I've ever heard from anyone." Now I was starting to raise my voice, and I told her in my sternest, loudest tones, "You will never, ever speak to me like this again. If you really want to see me, you will respect who I am and you will deal with that." I told her, "Leave this room right now, then knock on the door, come back in, and introduce yourself."

When she walked out, I wasn't sure she was going to come back, but she turned around and did exactly as I asked. What she needed was someone to set boundaries for her, and when I did, she became a different patient. She went from being a patient who was on the verge of hospitalization to one who was ready for recovery. Meanwhile, out in the waiting area, the other patient had seen the picture rampage and heard my raised voice. She said to my assistant, "Does he always yell at his patients like that?" And then she left. It was weeks before she made another appointment.

Today Hannah is one of my favorite patients—she's well on the road to recovery. Once the boundaries were set and she found someone who was able to stand up to her resistant attitude, she settled down and was ready to begin the real work of healing. Patient after patient has taught me that if you set the boundaries honestly in the beginning and deal with the patient with the same respect you're asking back, it works. Hannah and I are really straight with each other, and I think it goes back to that first session. She wanted someone who was strong enough to deal with her, and I showed her right away that I was up to the challenge and willing to help.

## The Therapeutic Process

A major part of the therapeutic aspect is to help patients understand that they're not ever going to get rid of some of the negative feelings they have. They don't have to get rid of them—they can live with them. It's how they adapt to them that matters.

As part of the therapeutic process, I ask my patients to define what their needs are in the real world. Individuals with eating disorders often take on too much. They don't know how to set limits or create boundaries and they tend to overstimulate themselves. What they're really doing is keeping so busy that they don't have time to deal with their underlying issues. They think they've got everything under control, and to outside observers, it looks like they do, at least on the surface. But they don't. They're doing a juggling act with their identity, basing it on approval from outside sources. Ask them who they're doing all this for, and they don't have a clue. Nobody can keep up a juggling act forever, and eventually things start crashing to the ground.

This is where the passion comes in. If they have a passion for something in life, if they have a focal point, they can deal with anxiety and other negative emotions. Understanding that they don't have to please every single person in the outside world and that they don't have to be perfect at every single thing they do gives them the freedom to pursue their own passions.

# Applying PIRT

Therapy for an eating disorder can be a long, slow, often difficult process. From the patient's perspective, it takes trust, patience, honesty, and faith that it will eventually work. From the therapist's perspective, it takes trust, patience, honesty, and faith that it will eventually work, along with a deep understanding of the issues that lie beneath the eating disorder. PIRT provides a basic framework for making the overall therapy as effective and valuable as possible.

SEVEN

# The Process of Recovering the Self

*Recovering from an eating disorder* is a slow and gradual process. As a patient moves toward recovery, in time, changes can occur. The individual may start to talk more openly about the eating disorder and the feelings attached to it. He may also start to change his point of view about it, becoming less defensive. In time, he'll begin to share more of his personal passions and interests and will move away from wanting to talk only about body image, food, the numbers on the scale, and the eating disorder label. But recovering from an eating disorder is rarely straightforward, and the path is never smooth. Just about all patients will experience slips, lapses, relapses, and even collapses. It's all part of the process of finding the self again.

## Defining Recovery

It's important to understand what recovery from an eating disorder involves. First, recovery does not mean that an individual's weight has returned to normal, either by weight gain or weight loss. In fact, in many ways weight is the last standard to use for judging recovery. Someone with anorexia, for instance, could regain all the lost weight but might still

---

*When the grip of the eating disorder loosens, then the individual's own self can take over again, leading to ultimate recovery: regaining your self.*

---

be just as depressed and anxious as before. To me, patients are in the process of recovery when they are eating in a more balanced way and their weight is stabilized for an extended period of time, when they are willing to try new foods and no longer have "fear foods" that must be avoided at all times. Symptoms of bingeing and/or purging, if those were issues, are no longer present on a continuous basis.

Recovery centers around the ability to cope with anxiety and depression and move forward through life's many stressors without a return to the eating disorder—or without substituting some other form of addictive behavior. Of course, there's no such thing as an absolute in recovery, no specific point at which to say, "Aha! This patient is now officially getting cured." Recovery isn't the absolute destination we'd like it to be. Sure, it involves physical progress, but it also involves personal and emotional healing. Generally speaking, a patient can be considered to be moving toward recovery when she starts talking positively about the concept of getting well, regarding it as something both desirable and attainable. It's important to understand, however, that wellness doesn't mean a return to all those high expectations. True wellness—and ultimate recovery—focuses on healing physically, emotionally, and spiritually, a coming together that makes the individuals feel reconnected to themselves again or for the first time.

## The Honeymoon Period

A patient may experience a honeymoon period when the eating disorder behavior is diminished to less activity and there's a significant improvement in medical stabilization. The family, the patient, and even the ther-

*Moving toward recovery can itself cause anxiety.*

apist exhale and think the worst is over. Unfortunately, that's often not the case. The biggest mistake for any patient to make is to stop treatment once the weight normalizes and they convince others "I'm fine now." I have had many patients leave therapy at that point, and I've had parents remove their child from treatment as soon as their child's out of immediate physical and emotional danger. No matter what the reason, when therapy stops too soon, the possibility of relapse, or collapse, increases dramatically.

Sometimes the honeymoon period actually causes anxiety in the patient. After a time of positive therapy and honest interaction in which she starts to feel a lot better about herself, a patient may start to think, "I'm getting better way too fast and that really scares me."

At that point, the individual may experience a slip or a lapse—a brief return to the eating disorder thoughts or behaviors. However brief, it can be very upsetting to the patient, who views it as a major setback. It's as if her mind is playing a game with her. In the struggle to get out of the eating disorder mind-set, a patient can feel she has failed if she engages in negative thoughts and behaviors.

# Setbacks and Stumbling Blocks

After years of treating individuals with eating disorders, I've found that the stumbling blocks along the way to recovery fall into four basic categories: slips, lapses, relapses, and collapses (see the chart on page 132). It's very common—in fact, I would call it normal—for individuals with eating disorders to experience at least the first two of those phases. In each phase, she is falling back into the safe haven of the eating disorder self.

## Slip

A slip is a thought—but not an action—related to the eating disorder. A slip is more than a return to thinking about the disorder or even contemplating the idea of perhaps skipping a meal or eating more than a normal portion. A slip is a thought that originates in the irrational, eating disorder mind and is closely related to actively participating in the eating disorder behavior. Someone who is anorexic, for instance, might find herself constantly thinking about food in a negative way and having negative feelings about her body, with increased thoughts of restricting her eating. Her thinking might go something like this: "I'm not going to eat that. It's going to make me fat. I have to start cutting down now." Someone who's bulimic might have overwhelming feelings of free-floating anxiety that lead to thoughts about bingeing and purging. Here the thinking goes along the lines of "I can't believe I ate all that. I'm so fat." Or "I feel so stuffed right now. I need to get rid of this food." And someone with binge eating disorder might start to feel very uncomfortable in her own skin, with strong feelings of emptiness and loneliness that lead to thoughts of bingeing to fill the emotional void. The thinking here is more like "I just don't know how to stop. And I'm so fat, what difference does it make if I eat it all?"

Every patient has slips, because every patient is human. Individuals with eating disorders can be incredibly hard on themselves, allowing their perfectionism to override their rational thoughts. They often think that one little slip means they have failed completely.

When a patient tells me about a slip after weeks of doing well, my usual response is that it is a normal occurrence. Their usual response is something like "You mean this was supposed to happen?" or "You mean it's okay to slip?" I reply, "I never expected you to be perfect." What I'm telling them is that true perfection is the ability to accept our own imperfections. "The key right here is not to allow the behavior to continue. You can stop it right now." To a perfectionist and obsessive person, one slip can mean a slide into the failure dynamic that may lead to a devastating

*True perfection is the ability to accept our own
imperfections.*

collapse. Some people take slips so personally and feel so guilty that they
may decide to reinvest in their illness. It's the therapist's goal to empower
these patients to give themselves permission to move forward.

Slips happen all the time. This is where trust in the therapist comes
in, because the patient does best if she talks with her therapist about the
slips rather than keeping them to herself. If a patient doesn't share the
occurrences, the thoughts just mount up, becoming so powerful and negative that she may not want to admit to them. The internal pressure of
hiding the slips can lead to a lapse, a sudden cascade of returning symptoms. The irrational mind shifts to irrational behaviors.

## Lapse

A lapse is more serious than a slip in that it moves beyond obsessive
thoughts and back into the eating disorder behavior, but in a limited way.
Although a lapse means the eating disorder behavior has become active
again, the experience is brief. It might involve just one or two episodes of
binge/purge behavior, for instance, rather than a larger pattern of the behavior over several days or longer. In the case of someone who has a pattern of bulimia, the lapse might be purchasing the binge food that triggers
the purging behavior. This action may create internal pressures that lead
to a return of the eating disorder behavior. I once had a patient with exercise bulimia who had a very rigid seven-day cycle of ritualistic exercise.
He was eventually able to stop the behavior, but when we first began
therapy he could only moderate it for a few months at a time. He would
lapse back into the exercise pattern for three or four weeks, but pull himself out of it each time.

---

*A lapse can be a common response to change.*

---

Lapses are generally short-term behavior—they don't necessarily mean a return to recurrent eating disorder behavior, but the irrational side of a patient's personality may magnify the lapse into a total failure. My patients will tell me that they have screwed up, just like they thought they would. The lapse makes them feel as if they've already blown it and might as well just give up. They can see only the failure and the guilt.

To help my patients get a better perspective on lapses, I first make them recognize how common the behavior is. Many of my patients can relate well to stories of what other patients have gone through—the stories make them feel less alone in their own behavior.

## Brian's Story

Brian was well into recovery, to the point that when he was offered a good job in another state, he decided to make the move even though it meant leaving therapy. The job was challenging enough, but moving away from family and friends to a place where he really didn't know anybody was an extra challenge. On top of that, Brian decided to take some extra courses at night toward a master's degree. All those transitions, all those new things at once created a lot of anxiety. When Brian needed someone to talk to about the anxiety, there wasn't anybody close by. As his anxiety level mounted, Brian started thinking more and more about the idea of returning to his old pattern of bulimic behavior. Suddenly, the eating disorder was again a way to cope with anxiety, and Brian couldn't resist it. He lapsed back into bulimia. However, Brian wasn't deeply invested in his eating disorder. He was able to realize that the lapse was in response to overwhelming stress, and he was able to decide for himself that this wasn't a place he wanted to stay.

Brian's lapse was brief and frightening, but when he was able to pull himself out of it, he realized that the lapse also showed him how far he had come. He took some steps to reduce his anxiety level by dropping one course and no longer volunteering for overtime at his job. He also found a therapist who could help him make the transition to his new environment more easily. Brian calls me now and then to check in. He's had more than a few slips and even another brief lapse, but overall he's doing extremely well.

To help patients cope with a lapse, I try to teach them how to process their feelings and to identify what triggers their key emotions. Transitions can leave people feeling empty and with a need to fill that void again with the eating disorder; a lapse can be a common reaction to change. My goal is to help them see that even if it doesn't feel that way while they're happening, lapses are almost always quick and short-lived. I also help patients get past their perfectionism and realize that a lapse isn't the end of the world, or an indication of total failure. I point out that there's no way anyone gets through recovery without slips and lapses. What's important is to recognize the lapse, work out of it, and allow self-forgiveness. I encourage my patients to talk about what happened and what triggered the behavior and discuss their thoughts of self-blame. I help them ask themselves, "What did I get from the lapse?" and answer the question honestly. We also talk about what they did to get over the lapse—what worked and what didn't—and how they can use the experience to get back onto the wellness path.

## Relapse

Far more serious, a relapse involves recycling the same eating disorder behavior that brought the person into treatment. A relapse means the behavior has returned on a regular basis, not just as an episode. It may even return to full intensity.

The difference between a lapse and a relapse is the difference between a stumble and a bad fall. When you stumble, you can catch yourself in the midst of it; when you fall, you can't stop yourself at all. A relapse means the patient is back into the illness for an extended period of time. Someone with anorexia, for instance, begins once again to restrict intake and limit food choices; someone with bulimia will binge and purge in the same pattern as before treatment; someone with binge eating disorder begins to gain weight from their nightly binges.

Relapses are almost always triggered by a significant change or transition in the individual's circumstances, such as changes in academic or professional status, leaving home to start college or a new job, altered personal relationships, or perhaps the death of a loved one. A relapse can also be triggered by an internal event, by which I mean an episode of depression or sometimes even recovery itself.

# Taylor's Story

Taylor was a gymnast who decided to increase his exercise routine as a way to improve his strength and performance. He did get stronger and his coach felt his performance was improved. This sort of positive outcome encouraged Taylor to extend his training, to the point where he eventually developed exercise bulimia.

As Taylor increased his exercise periods, however, he began to feel more and more pain in his ankles. At first he ignored the pain and worked through it, but it only intensified. He was finally diagnosed with stress fractures from overexercising. A perfectionist, Taylor refused to give up on his passion for gymnastics. But by not reducing his exercise level, he damaged his ankles even more and wasn't able to compete. At the same time, his compulsive overexercising (exercise bulimia) was actually making him weaker, not stronger.

Taylor finally sought treatment for his eating disorder so that he could remain a competitive gymnast. After months of treatment, his overall health and strength were improved enough that he could return to a modified training program. His long layoff and the damage to his ankles meant that he couldn't return to his previous level of excellence. Although his health was improved, Taylor's overall reaction to the situation was anger and despair—he felt he was a total failure. His core emotions led him to abruptly stop all his treatments: medical care, physical therapy, and psychotherapy. His own internal trigger let his irrational mind take over again and lead him into recycling his earlier eating disorder behavior. Here was a patient I thought was improving nicely, and yet the improvement itself turned into the trigger for a relapse.

Some patients are more prone to relapse than others. Generally speaking, the more often a patient has relapsed, the more likely it is to happen again. In these cases, changing the learned pattern of recovery/relapse is an important part of treatment. These patients can get frozen in place, fearing that any change in any direction will trigger a relapse.

I work with my patients to explore the triggers that have led to previous relapses and the methods that were most helpful in coming out of them. First on the list of things that can help is the community that is available to the patient. We look at the immediate and extended family, the patient's network of friends and peers, and also less obvious individuals such as pets, teachers, caretakers, spiritual/religious advisors, or work colleagues. By helping the patient see, in a rational way, that a significant support system is in place, I can help lower her anxiety about relapsing.

We also talk about the activities the patient has used in the past to replace the eating disorder, as well as activities that might interest her now. Building on an existing passion or finding a new one is an excellent way to break the relapse pattern and often helps the patient recognize that there's a distinct alternative to relapsing.

## Collapse

A collapse is the full-blown return of the original eating disorder behavior. An untreated relapse can turn into a collapse, and an untreated collapse can turn into an even more intense form of the illness, to the point that intervention and possibly hospitalization become necessary. Some-one in collapse not only may be experiencing the consequences of the eating disorder but may also be severely depressed or even suicidal.

Patients in collapse are no longer interested in a wellness identity—they have collapsed back into the eating disorder identity. They're fully engaged in the behavior and are justifying it to themselves and to every-one else.

Collapses generally occur in people who have had the illness for a significant period of time, but not always. Many have been through more than one cycle of relapse or collapse. When they're at the bottom of the abyss, and they're often there for a long time, beginning to climb out is extremely frightening, especially when the voice of the eating dis-order is still very much apparent. During this tentative period, they'd rather abandon the effort and justify staying in the disorder. These

# Four Phases of Declining into
# the Eating Disorder Self

| Slips | *Thoughts* <br> Based in the irrational mind |
|---|---|
| Lapses | *Behaviors* <br> Eating disorder becomes active again for a short period of time |
| Relapses | *Recycled Actions* <br> Recycling of prior eating disorder actions usually caused by external or internal triggering events |
| Collapses | *Full-Blown Illness* <br> Completely engaged in the eating disorder |

patients tend to engage and disengage with the illness. They'll have frequent episodes of active eating disorder behavior, but when the situation starts to get dangerous to their health, treatment intervention is necessary. Unfortunately, at that point the disorder is now controlling them. This is where the disease completely disables the desire to engage with wellness and may cause medical instability, severe depression, and suicidal thoughts.

# Handling Setbacks

Slips and worse, to the point of total collapse, tend to occur just when things seem to be finally going well in the patient's life. I have one patient, Alice, who seemed to be well on the way to getting over her anorexia. Her life was back on track and she was engaged—and then she found herself restricting her food intake again. She couldn't understand why she was being so self-destructive and felt very angry with herself. When we talked about it, Alice realized that for the first time in her life, everything was going well. That was so unfamiliar to her that dealing with it caused her more anxiety than she could imagine. She felt her life now was just too good to be true, that all the positive things that were happening to her would come crashing down sooner or later. That scared her. She felt it would be better to be in control of the crash when it happened, as she felt certain it would. At the same time, she was so accustomed to having a lot of really bad things in her life that she was unconsciously trying to turn the present good situation into a bad one. Bad is bad, of course, but it can also be reassuring and predictable.

*Many individuals with eating disorders don't feel they deserve to have good things happen to them. That's why, when things start going well, slips and lapses are likely to occur.*

This is a familiar pattern. Many individuals with eating disorders would rather return to a bad situation than stay in a good one. They believe they can control the bad situation through the eating disorder, but they don't have any idea how to handle a situation that's good. They also don't feel they deserve to have good things happen to them. That's why, when things start going well, slips and lapses are likely to occur.

The first thing I ask a patient when a slip occurs is "Why do you think this happened? What do you think triggered it?" We'll discuss the reasons behind the slip, and often the patient will tell me she's very angry with herself for her "failure." Individuals with eating disorders tend to see things in absolute, black-and-white terms. What I see as a minor slip, they see as a total failure. What I see as an opportunity to gain greater self-knowledge, they see as a reason to go deeper into despair.

When my patients slip up, I tell them that I know how they feel, because I, too, used to criticize myself for minor mistakes—and even for things that weren't mistakes at all, but just weren't as perfect as I wanted them to be. I encourage my patients to use a rational approach to help them understand that their all-or-nothing response is way out of proportion. I point out that nobody, especially me, expects them to be perfectly abstinent all the time and never have any slips. There's no need to beat yourself up so much, because the only person who expects you to never have a slip is yourself. I use the slip as a good example of how you can trip yourself up with your own perfectionism. I also use these moments to show them that setbacks are a normal part of life—they're simply part of the human condition.

---

*Individuals with eating disorders tend to see things in absolute, black-and-white terms. What someone else may see as a minor slip or an opportunity to gain greater self-knowledge, they see as a total failure, a reason to go deeper into despair.*

---

# Understanding Triggers

What's more important than blaming yourself for screwing up is understanding the trigger—the stressful or disturbing event—that caused the slip in the first place.

Some triggers are very obvious because they are related to emotional stress. Transitions are major triggers, as the story of Alice shows. Stressful events, such as a big exam or job interview, can also be triggers. Failure (not getting the job, for instance) is another big trigger. So is interpersonal strife: family arguments, breaking up with a boyfriend, divorce (a type of transition). Death of a loved one, another type of major transition, is a huge trigger—the loss of a parent, grandparent, spouse, or child, for instance. Even more positive things, like graduation, promotions at work, marriage, and pregnancy can be triggers, because even positive events can be stressful and can create anxiety. When anxiety is high, retreating back into the eating disorder identity is one way to handle it.

## Rachel's Story

My patient Rachel had been doing well for a long time; so long, in fact, that she had stopped needing therapy. I was surprised when she called and asked to see me again because she felt she was returning to her old eating disorder identity. When we met, I asked her if there was anything new going on that was causing this setback. She said there wasn't, but her depressed appearance and inability to look at me told me otherwise. I said, "Okay, Rachel, please step outside your box and look inside. What do you see?"

"I'm scared. A few weeks ago I found out I was pregnant," she said. I knew the pregnancy had to be unplanned. Rachel had been married for only a year, and I knew from past sessions she had been hesitant about having children right away.

Rachel knew that becoming a mother at this point in her life wasn't

*Transitions can be major triggers, as can stressful events such as interviews or arguments. Even positive events can be stressful and create anxiety. And when anxiety is high, retreating back into the eating disorder identity is one way to handle it.*

a good idea for her, but she felt it would be selfish to say so. Her husband wanted children. In addition, although Rachel and her husband were open with each other and he knew a lot about her, she had never told him that she had struggled with an eating disorder when she was a teenager. Now, at age twenty-nine, her pregnancy was creating a great deal of inner conflict and emotional stress and had triggered her eating disorder to return. This was a trigger on top of a trigger.

We had a long discussion about how the most important thing Rachel needed to relearn was what things were going to make her healthier, not what things she needed to do for other people. Right now she really needed to put her own needs first. That's not a selfish thing to do. She had to be honest with her husband and tell him of her past eating disorder and how the pregnancy was creating a serious risk to her at this point in her recovery. She needed to create an environment that was supportive, which in this case meant going back into treatment.

When Rachel revealed her eating disorder to her husband, he was very supportive. He realized that although Rachel had been in recovery for a long time, the transition of being pregnant had been a trigger for her. He understood how fragile she was. Once Rachel no longer felt under pressure about disclosing her past, she became open to continuing treatment through the course of her pregnancy. She quickly began to recover, had a normal pregnancy, and delivered a healthy, beautiful baby.

## Some Old Familiar Triggers

Gender identity issues can set up triggers. When patients who are uncertain or confused about their gender identity get called names, for instance, the experience can be a major trigger. Another trigger can be lost memories of trauma that resurface. This can happen in therapy, but it can also happen just in daily life.

Another common personal trigger is being with other people who have eating disorders. Being around the eating disorder behavior can trigger the behavior all over again. It seems to bring out the competitive juices of some of my patients—they think they have to be better at the disorder than the others. One of my patients, Cassie, is well into recovery, to the point where she's comfortable with giving talks on eating disorders to high school classes. But when a school counselor asked her to talk one-on-one with a young student who had anorexia, Cassie hesitated. Much as she wanted to help this young woman, she also knew that the conversation had real potential to be a trigger for her. With regret, she decided to say no. When we talked about this afterward, Cassie felt guilty about not helping. I pointed out that she should feel proud of herself instead. The young woman would still get help through her school counselor, and Cassie had avoided a dangerous situation. She had given up the caretaker role that was part of her eating disorder and had learned to articulate and act on her own needs.

Social eating—a meal out with family or friends—can also be a major personal trigger. The patients know that everyone knows about their eating disorder, which can make them feel as if everyone in the whole restaurant is watching them to see what they order and if they eat it. The self-consciousness and awkwardness of the situation can act as a trigger. On top of that, patients can make the situation worse and create their own triggers. Going to a steak house, being overwhelmed by the menu, and ordering only a salad with the dressing on the side, for example, only calls attention. In a situation like that, it's almost impossible for someone else not to say something about your choice. You've set yourself up for the response and created a trigger for yourself by making the situation very uncomfortable.

For many individuals, a particular food such as a rich dessert can be a trigger. The individual starts by thinking, "I'll just have a bite," and then eats the whole dessert. The guilt can trigger a cycle of bingeing and purging. I help my patients desensitize themselves to the trigger foods. I'd rather have them learn to cope than avoid the food completely, because I don't want my patients to be controlled by food. I ask them to imagine how they'll feel after they eat a portion of the particular food. If they think they can handle how they'll feel, I tell them to go ahead and eat. If they can't imagine themselves eating only a normal portion, or if they imagine themselves then purging, then that food still needs to be avoided.

## Transition as Trigger

The situations that set up the cascade of slip, lapse, relapse, and collapse almost always involve transition and change. Sometimes the situation is genuinely traumatic, such as a serious illness, death, or divorce in the family. More often the transition is something that many people would see as neutral or positive: graduation, starting college, a new job, engagement or marriage, the birth of a child. The common factor is the transitional events, negative or positive, that are part of ordinary life.

For many of my patients, any sort of change means changing expectations and living up to a higher standard. Starting a marriage, for instance, is a big change that brings challenges to everyone. For most people, the commitment of marriage is an important milestone, a positive event that is looked forward to with pleasurable anticipation, but for the individual with an eating disorder, who's a real perfectionist with a strong need to have everything under control, this becomes a setup for relapse.

If a positive transition can be so upsetting, negative transitions are even worse. Losing a job, having someone associated with a past trauma reenter your life, having a relationship break up, having a car accident—

these are all upsetting at the best of times. For someone recovering from an eating disorder, the intense anxiety of the event can be a trigger to relapse.

Another major trigger, paradoxically, can be transitioning back into normal life as part of recovery. I see this with individuals who have been so ill that they've had to withdraw from school, work, or just day-to-day living and are now trying to return to real life. The abrupt transition from isolation back into the chaotic realities of everyday life can be very difficult. Everyone assumes that because you're back into life again, you're fine. The reality is that while you're probably better, at least in terms of your weight and overall health, you still need support to negotiate the transition back into the real world. Without support—and sometimes even with it—a relapse can occur.

Transitions can leave someone feeling out of control—the ideal condition for a relapse or even collapse. Falling back into the eating disorder is a way to gain a sense of control rather than feeling swept away by all the change. Part of recovering from an eating disorder is getting better at handling change, whether it's negative or positive. When I talk about changes in their lives with my patients, we discuss good ways to deal with them. We work on ways for them to express themselves directly, rather than retreating back into the eating disorder behavior. I do role-playing with some of my patients, helping them work out in advance what their response to a potentially upsetting situation could be. And when a transitional situation doesn't go well, we look at it to see if the patient has unconsciously—or even consciously—set herself up for failure or self-sabotage.

# Expression of Self

George Bernard Shaw once said, "Life isn't about finding yourself. Life is about creating yourself." I often mention this to my patients when they've reached the point of transitioning away from their eating disorder. They no longer attach eating disorder behavior to the triggers, transitions, and traumas of their lives. Instead, they've developed healthier means of coping. I try to become a teacher, not a therapist, at this point. I explain that the metamorphosis from someone with an eating disorder to someone who is healthy can be painful, but that the struggle will be worthwhile. The self-knowledge they gain will allow them to have a solid chance for recovery and let them regain their true self. At this point, they have a choice about how they want to live their life: whole or self-defeated.

# EIGHT

# The Passion Pursuit

*Truly letting go* of an eating disorder means leaving a safe place to face life's transitions and challenges directly. That's not easy to do. It takes a lot of courage and determination—and it also takes learning to ask for help.

That's where therapy comes in. It's important for a therapist to help his or her patients discover new, healthier ways to handle anxiety and cope with change and transition; most of all, to help them discover who they are by locating the things they care about. Leaving behind the identity of an eating disorder means finding something to fill the void once dominated by obsessive concerns about eating, food, body image, and exercise. Individuals working to break free from the tangle of eating disorders need to find their passion in life. The goal is to shift the focus from destroying the self to enhancing the self, and to transition away from the eating disorder identity. There are much healthier channels for the energy once put into their eating disorder. The challenge is to find them.

## Filling the Void

The passion pursuit is a fundamental aspect of my approach to treating patients with eating disorders. By passion I mean something external that gives the individual enjoyment, positive structure, or a pathway to self-knowledge. That's not easy, though, because almost all of my patients are so wrapped up in their eating disorder that they can barely imagine their lives without it. I am not suggesting an immediate swap of one for another, but a gradual replacement.

Many individuals with eating disorders have never been asked about any aspect of their life outside of their weight and their eating disorder symptoms. For some, the question is so unexpected that they can't even really understand it at first. But I have yet to find someone who doesn't, deep down, have some sort of real interest in something. My patients all have interests and passions; they've just suppressed them or never been given the opportunity to discover them.

# Structure and Ritual

The person with a serious eating disorder has no time in their life for anything other than obsessing about the next meal, overexercising, and perfectionist rituals. That doesn't leave any space for fun. That doesn't even leave any idea of what fun is. What others might see as time for fun and relaxation, they see simply as nonproductive time that has to be filled with obsessive activity.

At this point in an eating disorder, to a large extent, patients' minds aren't their own, and they simply can't grasp the idea of having fun or enjoying something that's not within the parameters of their eating disorder. Any outside interests would only distract their focus, which would be a scary proposition.

*To someone with an eating disorder, trying something new means disrupting the ritualized structure. Anything that alters the rules of the game or breaks the rituals that make up his day is upsetting or panic-inducing.*

The person with an eating disorder tends to be very fearful of new things—she doesn't like change. To her, something that rocks her world is more like rocking her boat. And why explore something new when you can stay safely inside the rituals and compulsive behavior of your eating disorder? Most people think that trying something new is fun, or at least different—a way to break up the monotony of everyday life. To someone with an eating disorder, however, trying something new means disrupting the structure she has created for herself. Anything that alters the rules of the game or breaks the rituals that make up her day is upsetting or panic-inducing. Those rituals are what she uses to control her world, and anything that makes her feel she's losing control is dangerous and terrifying.

## The Control Box

I try to get my patients to realize that they're trapped in a box of their own making and encourage them to look beyond that box. That's hard at first. Ask someone with an eating disorder to describe what their box looks like, and you'll get answers that are rigidly defined by ritual. The box is very symmetrical, it's got sharp, square corners, it's black-and-white, and it doesn't have any openings. It has no light inside it, no atmosphere, and very little escapes from it. That sort of box is colorless and uncreative—it's more of a fortress than anything else—but staying in that existing, well-defined box means staying in control.

To get patients started on ways to move out of that control box, I sometimes ask them to describe their daily routine to me. A patient may tell me, "I get up at five in the morning and exercise on the treadmill for thirty minutes and then take a morning run outside for sixty minutes. Then I eat breakfast at 7:05, then I take a shower and get dressed and leave for work at 8:10." If I ask, "What if you planned to exercise in the evening instead?" her eyes will bulge and I can almost hear her thinking, "Are you out of your mind?" Most patients are too polite to say that and instead will give me long rationales for their morning routine and why they couldn't possibly change it. One big reason for resisting change is that it would mean altering their entire schedule. For many eating disorder

---

*Most people with eating disorders have very rigid schedules.
Extreme distress over a seemingly minor change in
routine is typical.*

---

patients, schedules are extremely important. Any alteration or disruption gets them extremely agitated.

One of my patients, Abbey, arrived for her session in a state of near hysteria. Her father was running late that day and couldn't get home in time to prepare her evening meal and have it ready at precisely 6:30 PM. Instead, her father told her, "We'll just take the food with us and you can eat it in the car on the way to the doctor's office." Abbey lost it! Her whole day was structured around eating a specific set of foods, prepared by a specific person, in very specific amounts, at a very specific time and place. Instead, she would have to eat the food in a different place and with a time limit. She couldn't handle it. Their entire drive to my office was nothing but a screaming match between Abbey and her father, and the food ended up being thrown all over the car, all over Abbey, and all over her father. It was pretty clear to me just from Abbey's appearance what had happened, but I spent most of the session calming her down enough for her to tell me, in her own words, how the change in schedule affected her.

Abbey's extreme distress over a seemingly minor change in her routine is typical for someone with an eating disorder. Many individuals with eating disorders get fixated on particular foods and will eat little else. They'll insist on preparing the food in exactly the same way, having exactly the same portion, and eating it in exactly the same place at exactly the same time. The rigidity can be extreme, and it often gets worse as the weight goes dramatically up or down and the obsessive behavior takes over even more. The eating rituals tend to repeat themselves and get even more involved and complex.

The same thing happens with compulsive overexercising, also known as exercise bulimia. The same exercises have to be done in the same sequence at the same time every day. Instead of becoming more restrictive over time, however, the exercise becomes more elaborate. If the ritual calls for thirty minutes on the exercise bike one day, it will call for thirty-two minutes the next day. Calories become the inverse of exercise. As the ritual gets more complicated and the exercise patterns increase, the calories go down and the exercise goes up.

# Exploring Interests

As part of my initial assessments with patients, I attempt to find things that have the potential to interest them. I almost always get hints of new areas we can explore or get a glimpse of an earlier passion that has been submerged under the eating disorder. What I then try to do is build on those early hints and work with the patient to find and develop the passion. What I'm hoping to do is not simply trade one type of obsessive behavior—the eating disorder—for another that's less physically harmful. If all I do with the patient is swap one set of obsessions for another, the chances are good that the eating disorder will reassert itself sometime down the road. I want my patients to find their passions but also to integrate those passions into real life. I want them to use their passion not just inwardly, filling the void left by the eating disorder, but in external ways within their families, their communities, their lives as fully functioning individuals.

Going back to school is a good way to begin. Many of my patients have had their educations seriously disrupted by their illness. In their minds, school is associated with failure and trauma. Some have been put on medical leave from high school or college; some have simply dropped out; others have been asked to withdraw. Some were labeled as learning disabled but never got the extra help they needed to use their intelligence and succeed academically. Others were excellent students but were driven by perfectionism. These patients experienced school as the place where they crashed and burned, but also as a place where they excelled. Others were good students whose academic ambitions were frustrated by family disapproval or pressure.

Patients are often taken out of school—the logic being that school is a stressor and that removing the stressor is supposed to help the patient—and the schools support this approach, but more because removing the student removes liability issues. Interrupting someone's education like that is, in my opinion, often unnecessary. It leads to a tremendous amount of guilt and anxiety. There's often a lot of embarrassment and shame, because up until the moment the student drops out, she is totally unaware of the possible consequences, such as falling behind a grade or losing all her academic credits or not being allowed to return.

There are significant problems with removing someone from school. It often effectively ends the patient's education. Many will never go back; if they do, they'll have a hard time explaining where they were while they were out of school. Others will end up completing their degrees much later than their peers. Without school, they become isolated from their friends and community. Most damaging is that nothing fills the empty time once school is removed. For people with obsessive-compulsive tendencies and an eating disorder, empty time is the enemy. When there's little else to do, the eating disorder and OCD behavior can really blossom.

My philosophy is to try to never pull the patient out of school unless it's an absolute emergency. If a patient really must drop out, I try to be sure the right arrangements are made for a medical leave that keeps open the option to return. Most schools are fairly cooperative, because they have become more aware and understanding of these kinds of circumstances.

I don't want to protect my patients from life's stresses, I want them to learn to navigate within them. I'd rather keep them in the stressful environment and teach them how to cope with it.

I strongly encourage patients who are in school to stay there, and

---

*The goal is not to protect the individual from stresses, but to help them learn how to navigate within them.*

I encourage those who have dropped out without degrees to return. Part of this is purely practical—in today's society, a college degree is essential for any sort of meaningful employment. The larger reason, however, is that school is a place to find and pursue a passion that can become a career-driven pathway.

# Bette's Story

Bette came from a wealthy family with high expectations of her—she was expected to have the sort of career that was prestigious and highly paid. Despite a lack of real interest in the field, Bette dutifully went into real estate and hated every minute of it. She got married and continued to work, but the anxieties of work were overwhelming and the transition to being a wife became too much for her. Bette developed severe anorexia. After months of treatment, she finally admitted to me that when she was a teenager she had wanted to become some sort of therapist or school counselor—she wanted to do something with her life to help others. Her family had strongly discouraged her. The argument was "Why do you want to hear about other people's problems? There's no money in that. Go get yourself a real job."

Bette suppressed her own desires to live up to the expectations of her family. When I suggested the possibility of going back to school for the appropriate degree in counseling to become a therapist, she leaped at the idea. Somehow we had released an interest that had been dormant for years. The problem then became one of holding Bette back. In typical eating disorder fashion, she wanted to jump right in with a course load that would have crushed someone in much better physical and mental health.

Her course work became a passion for her—and the eating disorder decreased in intensity. Before she went back, all she could do was focus on her body. Week after week, all she had talked about was how fat she looked and how much she was eating. Her food rituals and poor health no longer fit with her new life as a graduate student. She had to choose either the eating disorder or school, and Bette chose school.

Bette has real enthusiasm for the intellectual challenge of her program and her future career. She's not just substituting a new obsession with school for the old food obsessions. Her new identity as a therapist-to-be is much stronger and more well grounded than her old identity as a person with an eating disorder. And once she rediscovered her passion, it gave her the strength to resist family disapproval for her choice. She was able to make them see that her new career might be less financially rewarding but was much more satisfying to her than her former identity.

# Megan's Story

Sometimes all it takes is for the therapist to validate the old passion and "allow" the patient to return to it. One of my recent patients was a young woman who was a competitive dancer. Megan had always had a great passion for dance; from grade school through high school she had been a very talented dancer. Slimness is important in this activity, however, and when she was in college the pressure on Megan to keep her weight down eventually led her into bulimia. Because the bulimia made her anemic and caused other health problems, her physician advised her not to dance, saying it was too dangerous. Her therapist agreed, thinking that competitive college dancing was too stressful for her. What that led to was someone with bulimia who was now also extremely depressed. Dancing, the thing she loved most, had been taken away—and there was nothing but the bulimia to take its place. The enemy wasn't the dancing, the enemy was the empty space left when the dancing was taken away. It didn't take long after that for the eating disorder to become Megan's entire identity.

I asked Megan why she wasn't dancing anymore. She told me about the medical and therapeutic advice she had received, but I strongly suspected there was a lot more to it. As we talked more over several sessions, it became clear that the pressure of high-level competition wasn't the root cause of her bulimia. The real reason was the destructive breakup of her parents' marriage, a situation that left Megan's mother with a lot of anger and resentment. In some ways, Megan's illness was an attempt to reduce the family tensions by bringing her parents together again through their concern for her.

During our later sessions I told Megan I thought dancing again would be a very good idea for her, as long as she eased her way back into it. She looked at me in astonishment, then broke out into a big smile.

To get her dancing again safely, I referred her to forms of movement therapies, including yoga and Pilates classes. I wanted not only for Megan to take up her passion again but also for her to build up trust in her body and herself. My focus is on strengthening the center to strengthen the whole.

I was concerned about her health issues, and I knew she had the sort of personality that would lead her straight into overactivity if we weren't careful. At the time, I didn't know very much about competitive dancing. I've since learned a lot from Megan, as I am often taught by my patients through their passions.

I realized that we had to call in Megan's community. I started by calling Megan's trainer. He was wary at first. The trainer had seen Megan's talent, but he had also seen Megan at the height of her bulimia. He was concerned about the health issues and frankly didn't want to put up with any more liability. I told him that his concerns were perfectly valid. The difference now was that I was working with Megan to get the bulimia under control and that going back to dancing would be very therapeutic for her. I also told him I didn't want Megan getting totally involved too quickly, because she still needed to regain her weight and physical strength. This is the point when the passion becomes transitional, bringing the individual through illness into health.

The trainer and I talked about how to ease Megan back into dancing as safely as possible given her physical conditions. We decided she would start by dancing only once a week while also attending her other movement therapies, until her physical endurance improved. I used dancing as a sort of bait, a way to move Megan's focus away from her eating disorder and back toward a new goal. As the purging behavior became less frequent, she became physically stronger and was able to handle dancing more often.

I also spoke with Megan's university and the psychologist from their student counseling center about getting her back into classes for the next semester. They were reluctant at first, because Megan had missed so many days. Although she had been a good student in the beginning, as her bulimia got worse her grades had plummeted and she had become difficult to handle. Also, she had dropped out abruptly, without ever doing any of the paperwork to arrange a medical leave. Megan's parents had to attend a lot of meetings and complete a lot of paperwork to straighten out the situation with the school. That turned out to be a good thing, because it got her parents more involved in something tangible as a way to help their daughter.

A big reason the trainer and the school were willing to give Megan the benefit of the doubt and work with her again was that I told them how important they were to her recovery. My feeling is that the more help and support the patient has, and the more connected she feels to a larger community, the better. Often all you have to do to get the community involved is just ask.

I see Megan only once a month now as maintenance therapy. The change in her is remarkable. She's back to competitive dancing and she has graduated from college. Her ritualized behaviors of bingeing and purging as a way to cope have been out of her life for years.

Megan's dancing is an activity calling for a great deal of athleticism and a particular type of body image. It's not surprising that the pressure to be slender played a role in her eating disorder. Many sports, such as gymnastics, track, skating, and wrestling, put a premium on body image. They call for a slender, very toned body with no visible fat. For serious athletes, the pressure to be thin is enormous—and it often comes from their coaches. That pressure, combined with the same determination that makes these young people so good at their sport, can lead them into eating disorders as they strive for even better performance. As a therapist, I have to walk a very careful line in treatment. On the one hand, I want them to get well, but on the other, I want them to maintain their passion. What I don't want to do is reinforce the negative body image that played into the eating disorder.

# The First Step

The very idea that there might be something else out there beyond the eating disorder is a big step for any eating disorder patient. It can take a while for the lightbulb to go on—and when it does, the first thing the patient feels is the anxiety of something new. The awareness can become exciting, but processing it can be scary. Moving ahead from there can take a lot of time, because you have to walk with the patient through every step of the transition. Otherwise, there's a good chance they'll sabotage themselves without even realizing it. I start by making it real for them. We explore their anxieties and ask if each step makes sense to them. A big part of the awareness of the passion is that it has to be rational. I have to keep patients from going off the deep end. Someone who can't really function well in a competitive school situation, for instance, could still make an extreme choice and decide to try for a top college. That's just setting yourself up for failure. When you don't get in, your passion is beaten down and you feel rejected all over again. Unconsciously, my patients know their own capabilities and passions—they just need some help from me to discover them.

## Drew's Story

Age twenty-six when I first began to see him, Drew was anorexic, significantly underweight, and very concerned about his body image and gender identity. He was also very shut down—I could hardly get him to say a word in our early sessions. Drew's anxiety level was so high that he couldn't hold down a job anymore. That only made the eating disorder worse, because all he did was stay home and worry about food. Socially, Drew was extremely isolated. He didn't seem to have any friends and he hardly spoke to his family members. There didn't seem to be anyone or anything that interested him.

After months of regular sessions with me, I still didn't know much about Drew. Almost in desperation, I started talking to him about music. I asked him if he liked music and, if so, what sort. Just about everybody likes some kind of music, and Drew was no exception. He told me about some songs and bands he liked. When I thought about them, I realized they all had one thing in common—great guitar players. Drew liked the sound of the guitar. I took a chance and asked him, "Do you play the guitar?" His instant response was "I don't want to talk about it." I asked, "Why not?" and got the reply "I just don't want to talk about it." That told me I was getting close to something important, but I wanted Drew to tell me about it in his own time. Sure enough, after many months, he finally began to open up. What he told me was a story of being raped by a male music teacher. That certainly explained a lot about why Drew was so shut down, why he wasn't playing the guitar even though he was a talented musician, and why he was conflicted about his gender identity. Every time he picked up his guitar, a flashback of the horrible experience would come flooding back.

Before Drew's next scheduled session, I went out and bought a very inexpensive plastic guitar—a toy to visually represent to Drew what he had deleted from his life due to the trauma he had experienced. I gave it to Drew at the start of our next session, telling him, "In case you ever get interested again, this is just to remind you of the memories you had playing the guitar." He took it but didn't say anything. In that session and for several more months, music never came up. Then, to my surprise, Drew's mother called and told me he was playing the guitar again for the first time in months. Happy as his mother was to see Drew doing something he enjoyed again, she was also worried. Now that she understood Drew's tendency toward excessive behavior, she was concerned that he would practice too much. She was also concerned that he would revive his interest in music as a career, something she and the rest of the family strongly opposed.

I could see her point about overpracticing—Drew definitely could go in that direction. I also know from my other patients that people with eating disorders often have trouble setting limits for themselves. It's important to endorse a passion but set some boundaries at the same time. We agreed to set some limits for Drew in terms of when and for how long he would practice each day. Drew resented that, but I saw that as a positive thing. Every normal individual resents limits, but they actually want them.

We also set some other goals, the first being to get Drew back to taking lessons again. As for Drew's possible future as a professional musician, we'll see how far his talent takes him.

# Expressing Yourself

Some of my patients are lost when it comes to expressing their passions; they simply don't have the words to express how they feel. They've lost their voices. That's where I've found that two really valuable tools— creative arts and journaling—can become their voice.

I ask these patients to express their lost voice visually or in writing. The medium can be anything—a collage, a painting or drawing, a sculpture, a photograph, a poem, a play, or just a cluster of words and colors. It doesn't matter if the patient has any particular creative talent or not. What I want is something we can talk about as a way to unlock the patient's voice.

To help with the creative process, I give patients open-ended themes. I might suggest they create or write something that represents what they're experiencing. I ask questions such as "What does your identity look like?" or "What does your voice sound like?" or "What does your eating disorder look like?"

Rather than sitting across from the patient just talking in standard therapeutic language, or having those long periods of silence, we can talk through their creations. I can ask broader questions, like "What does this mean to you?" or "Imagine this isn't your work. Take a step back and tell me what you see." Often it's like breaking down a dam of silence. But there is usually some hesitation when the patient is first introduced into this process.

The same thing can happen when patients keep journals or do any other kind of writing, such as poetry or stories. Journaling, creative writing, and allowing patients to e-mail gives them a way to communicate indirectly and directly. Any form of communication that will give me a clearer picture helps with therapeutic communication. To better understand my patients, I sometimes ask them to read their journals aloud to me. This reconnects the patients to their own written words and lets their silent voice be heard. (If they're uncomfortable reading their own entries aloud, sometimes they'll ask me to read them on their behalf.)

Journal entries are extremely personal—the words can represent the individual's innermost feelings—and there has to be a lot of trust between the therapist and the patient before that sort of sharing can happen. In this example from a patient named Ellie, the struggle to give up the eating disorder identity is conveyed very powerfully:

> *Walking down a road I felt my body's strength, my confidence & courage toward struggles, and my passions for life. The traumas that once plagued me were held as past tense and I no longer claimed them as a security to restrict others from knowing my authentic self. As I exhaled, a voice of truth filled with feelings and hope was heard.*

> *On this walkway cracks slowly started to appear on the pavement, I recognized them but denied that they were breaking the foundation below. I walked slowly down the crumpling road and kept moving forward. I started to feel alone, overwhelmed, and imprisoned. I began to realize that the place I was in was not safe. I was caught up in the work of living and began to lapse into negative thoughts and feelings. I started to feel the effects of the past and the traumas, but realized I was not just feeling it I was reliving it. Caught in the darkness as the sun set, I did not know how to voice the word "help." I got too caught up in the silence of the darkness to reach out. So I faked the walk I was supposed to perform for others—emptied my spirit and filled it with more silence. The voice that once expressed feelings and hope was restricted by past*

secrets and isolation. The ground separated and the small cracks became a large gaping hole. I fell hard and fell fast, when I hit the ground I remembered this old familiar place and realized that the eating disorder I spoke about in past tense was now presently face to face with me. What more do I have to learn? What more do I have to heal from? What do I choose, a continous power struggle for wellness or a life of entrapment?

I feel shameful of where I am because I am supposed to be this powerful example of strength and I am currently nowhere near perfect. Residing in sickness that allows me to cope in a dysfunctional way. I want health, I want freedom, I want my life back, but I do not want to abandon the place I am in right now because I am in this space for a reason. I don't want to jump back into a falsified recovery for an external reason either. I want to finally choose my own reasons for staying and living in a recovered state of mind, body, and soul. I need to accept who I really am without the mask, I need to heal the layers that pull me back into painful moments surrounded by silence, and begin to embrace the power and success that come with health, recovery, and life.

I don't want to dwell in the darkness; I know I currently find myself there because I could no longer handle the surroundings, the destructions, the perfection, the expectations of others, the depression and anxiety that creates an overwhelming pressure, and being trapped in the past scenarios that I no longer want in my present.

I have been on this journey before, but this time I have to let go of the eating disorder or get dragged down. I get so angry toward myself when I let go of my voice instead, resulting in a shutdown mode of silence. I fear the work that is needed to find a way out, but I know the pain can be shared. Freedom can occur even if that will lead me into a transitional unknown, I don't want a life dictated by my own self-destruction!

Ellie's written words helped me understand why she had so much trouble saying anything in therapy. Her journal entries told me she had the words to express herself, but that she couldn't bring herself to actually say them aloud, even in the safety of a session. The written word helped her to organize her feelings and express them.

*My patient Haley* used her powerful writing skills to create a series of revealing dialogues—short plays, really—during her treatment. The dialogues were "conversations" between herself and her eating disorder. As we read them aloud, she would take the part of herself and I would play the role of her eating disorder. The dialogues were extremely revealing— what Haley expressed in them is exactly how many other individuals with eating disorders feel as well. This dialogue, for instance, captures very precisely the struggle many patients feel as they get ready to let go of their eating disorder identity:

SELF:    I don't need you anymore.

VOICE:   That's not true.

SELF:    Well, what makes you think I need you? What are you offering me?

VOICE:   A ticket out of every difficult situation that you don't want to be in. You know that's what you need.

SELF:    But you're not really offering me anything. It's just an illusion.

VOICE:   Yeah, right, an illusion. That's not what you've believed for all this time.

SELF:    I'm finally starting to believe what people I trust are telling me, not what you say. I'm getting scared from being here for so long.

VOICE:   They're just jealous. They'd rather be in your shoes any day.

SELF:    But I need to get my mind back. You've taken over my mind.

VOICE:   I didn't take it over—you gave me the key and asked me to stay. Now that outside people are creating some fears you want me out. Tough. I'm staying.

SELF:    You're just manipulating me now. I'm going to get worse if I keep listening to you.

VOICE:   No, you're going to become perfect, not worse. Why do you think you worked so hard at this? Was it for others or yourself? If your answer is for yourself you're a liar—it was for others.

SELF:    The pain is just getting so bad now.

VOICE:   That's the price for perfection. I thought you were so much stronger than this. I guess you're just as weak as they are.

SELF:    Those words are not going to work this time! I am not going to listen to you. I am going to break free from this eating disorder once and for all.

VOICE:   Sure you are. Who are you listening to right now? You're talking because I'm responding. You say you don't want to listen to me, but I bring you strength. You say you want to break free from an eating disorder, but that's the garbage others feed you. You don't really believe it.

SELF:    I'm stronger now than I was before, I have more support around me now. There are a lot of people who understand me now. I don't have to listen to just your voice any longer.

VOICE:   Well, where are they? All I see is you and me. I understand you better than anyone . . . I created you.

SELF:    Go away—leave me alone! I'm not going to let you win. You're the liar, not me. This worked in the past but it doesn't work now.

VOICE:   Oh, did I upset you? I'm so sorry, but think about it. Who are you without me?

SELF:    I don't know who I am without you yet, but I want to find out. I have to find out. I may not know who I am yet but I know there is more to me than you.

VOICE:   We're finally in agreement. I know there's more to you
         as well, but that's the side you use to cover me up.
         Remember, it's safer to keep me than to explore your past.

SELF:    You're repeating yourself again—you said this the last time
         we talked. It's the same old thing. You just want me to be
         dependent on you, and I feel like I've sold out to you long
         enough.

VOICE:   Yet we are here once again, still having the same
         conversation over and over. I think you're just too fearful
         to really say good-bye. Admit it, you still need me. You
         may not want me any longer but you need what I offer
         you—safety . . . understanding . . . commitment.

SELF:    Commitment? You're only committed to keeping me! You
         only want to keep me trapped. That's not commitment,
         that's imprisonment. You're right about my being scared,
         but you don't offer me any real safety. I'm getting sicker
         and weaker.

VOICE:   You, you, you! Poor you! You make it sound like I abuse
         you when in reality you've abused yourself all along. All I
         tried to do was support your efforts. I provided safety from
         the others who called you fat. I provided understanding as
         you buried your secrets. I provided commitment to you as
         a person. I believed in you when no one else did. If we're
         going to part ways, recognize this—I will always be a part
         of you.

SELF:    Maybe. I can live with that. It's okay with me if you're
         always a little part of me, just as long as you're not all of
         me.

I felt that Haley had achieved a real breakthrough with this dialogue. She captured the tug-of-war that goes on between the self and
the eating disorder and the inner conflict between wanting to be free
from the eating disorder and being afraid to be free.

Creative arts and writing are wonderful ways to express yourself, and they're also ways to relieve distress and decrease anxiety. These creative acts fill some of the space that's occupied by the eating disorder. It's also revealing, both to the patient and to me. It's sometimes easier to create something that can't be expressed by words alone. What my patients discover is that creative work can be therapeutic and enjoyable, even if it's also an "assignment." Many of these individuals have learned to use their therapeutic creativity as an ongoing form of self-therapy long after their therapy with me has been completed.

NINE

# Family and Community Identity

*Eating disorders* can destroy families—or bring them together. Bringing together the strengths of the individual and the family and community can mean all the difference in how well and how quickly a patient recovers from an eating disorder. How can family members and others learn to avoid destructive statements? How can they learn better ways to communicate? And how can they find ways to articulate and cope with their own feelings about the patient with the eating disorder?

For someone with an eating disorder, the support of the family and community can be invaluable, leading to a faster recovery. Teaching the family and the community the language of eating disorders is essential to help the patient shift away from the eating disorder identity. Family sessions and support groups that involve the family, friends, and community create more understanding and help remove the blame, shame, and guilt from the patient. With or without a highly supportive family and a community of caring people, however, recovery is rarely quick and easy. Setbacks happen as the patient gropes for a new identity.

# Family Impacts

Individuals with eating disorders come from every type of family—good, bad, indifferent—and every level of society. And yet, while no family is typical, over the years I have noticed some patterns that seem to be strongly associated with eating disorders.

A family history of eating disorders, addiction, general anxiety disorder, and obsessive-compulsive disorder is a common thread among many of my patients. We know from twin studies and recent genetic research that there's a hereditary element in eating disorders. We're still a very long way from knowing exactly why, how, or who, but it has been clear to me for a long time that family history can play a role by creating a tendency toward these disorders. When I ask a patient to construct a family tree, the incidence of disordered eating, alcoholism, drug addiction, and other addictions among immediate family members can be strikingly high. Time and again, as a patient starts to move into recovery, the mother or father may reveal to me that he or she experienced disordered eating (an abnormal form of eating behavior that is not a diagnostic entity), an eating disorder, or some other form of addictive behavior as an adolescent or young adult. Similarly, I sometimes find that a patient has a sibling who also had or has an eating disorder. That's not very surprising. Siblings share the same family setting and a lot of the same genes.

---

*Having a family history of eating disorders, addictions, and obsessive-compulsive disorder doesn't guarantee that someone will develop an eating disorder. It does suggest, however, that awareness of the possibility needs to be present, just as there needs to be an awareness of a family history of, say, breast cancer or diabetes.*

---

As well, if there's a major family problem such as one sibling with a serious illness, other siblings can get put on hold, and if the problem is an eating disorder, the other siblings learn that they can bring some attention back to themselves by getting one, too. This isn't a calculated move. They see the secondary gains of an eating disorder—the extra attention—and unconsciously come to the conclusion that this could have major benefits.

Having a family history of eating disorders, addictions, and obsessive-compulsive behaviors doesn't guarantee that someone will develop an eating disorder. It does suggest, however, that awareness of the possibility needs to be present, just as there needs to be an awareness of a family history of, say, breast cancer or diabetes.

Marital conflict is also a major factor. A disproportionate number of my patients with eating disorders come from single-parent homes or from families where the parents are in serious conflict (whether or not it's out in the open), separated, or divorced. Sometimes the eating disorder is an unconscious attempt to reunite the parents or defuse the tension by focusing the attention on the "sick" child. Usually, though, the eating disorder is an individual's way of coping with the severe anxiety caused by parental conflict.

Serious illness within the family is another contributing factor that I see among my patients. Sometimes a parent or grandparent is ill; sometimes it's another child in the family. While all the family attention is focused on the ill person, someone else in the family is quietly developing an eating disorder. On the surface it may seem as if the person with the eating disorder is just looking for more attention by making herself sick, but there's much more to it than that. What's really going on is that the illness in the family is creating a lot of anxiety. If an individual

---

*The eating disorder, with all its ritualistic behavior, can become a way to handle anxiety and stay in control.*

---

is also a perfectionist or tends toward obsessive-compulsive behavior, she may start to feel even more anxious as the normal routines are disrupted by the family illness. The eating disorder, with all its ritualistic behavior, becomes a way to handle the anxiety and feel more in control.

# Community Impacts

When I first started treating patients with eating disorders in the early 1970s, the problem was something to hush up and try to keep within a small circle of family members and close friends. While that's still the case in some families today, over the years eating disorders in women have been destigmatized to a remarkable extent. (Men with eating disorders are still very much stigmatized.) I think the difference is largely due to the increased number of female celebrities who acknowledge their struggle with an eating disorder on television and in the press. Pleased as I am to see a serious medical problem come out from the shadows, celebrities can make it seem as if an eating disorder is something relatively minor that you just somehow catch, like a bad cold. Glamour and fame can make eating disorders seem trendy, and even desirable, as if an eating disorder is something you can choose to have. Then, when they appear looking all happy and healthy again, they make it seem as if getting over the disorder is easy and that the illness has no lasting effects. Sadly, that's far from the truth.

## *The Danger of Group Identity*

In recent years I've seen a disturbing increase in the number of eating disorder groups among high school and college students. In this situation, young women within the school setting band together, almost like an informal club, and support one another in their eating disorder. They'll even wear different color bracelets to signify the differences between who is anorexic, who is bulimic, and who is both. They will all sit together in the cafeteria at lunchtime, for instance, and help one another get through that time without eating. They also form bingeing and purging groups, to teach each other to do it better and more often. These groups can be quite large, reaching a dozen or more members. When I've talked with young women who have participated in this sort of group behavior, what I've noticed is that before they found one another, they tended to be isolated and set apart, with few friends. Often the group starts when one individual develops an eating disorder and others are attracted to the idea. They find an identity in the eating disorder, but they also find something more. By joining the illness, they find friendship and community. Some can't stay with it—they don't like being hungry all the time or throwing up a lot—but others get sucked in and develop true eating disorders. The chemical changes that occur from restricting and purging can quickly become an addiction, and the eating disorder can get a firm grasp on the individual.

Eating disorder groups can arise in any situation that brings young women together. They're found in college dorms and sororities. The group members support one another in the illness. Their motto is "Don't give in, don't give up." By that, they mean don't give in to the desire to eat, don't admit that the eating disorder is a problem, and resist any attempt to treat it. Instead, claim it's a lifestyle choice and fight any effort to interfere with the decision. This is the same message and same support that people today can easily find online at pro–eating disorder websites, chat rooms, video blogs, and social networking sites, except it's live and in person.

---

*Some young women find identity among eating disorder groups where they band together, almost like an informal club, and support one another in their eating disorder.*

---

Being open about having an eating disorder sometimes makes it easier to deal with community response. If teachers and the school system (and that applies also to undergraduate and graduate college programs) know what the problem is, they can try to accommodate the situation. When someone just disappears from the school system with no explanation, getting one back in can be very difficult. When the school is kept fully informed, however, going on medical leave for an eating disorder becomes a real alternative to dropping out or being forced out. The school or college can make serious efforts to keep the student on track academically. Arrangements can be made to keep one in school part-time or with a home tutor; if the student needs to spend time in a residential program, the schoolwork done there can be coordinated with the home school curriculum. I've found that for most of my patients, the school or college system is eager to help. These students were usually academically stellar up until their illness forced a crash.

## The Celebrity Syndrome

When celebrities go on talk shows and disclose their struggles with eating disorders, it seems like all it took to "cure" them was a few sessions with a therapist or maybe a few weeks in a residential program. Some of the younger celebs make having anorexia sound almost like having a childhood illness—something you just get and get over, like chicken pox. They rarely talk about the misery they felt while in the grip of the eating disorder. They don't talk about the toilet bowls and the vomiting, the sickness and stomach cramps, the black rings under the eyes and the hair that falls out. All they talk about is how it's behind them, how great they look and feel now, and the exciting new project they're doing.

*Actors and models appearing on talk shows make it sound as if getting over an eating disorder is quick and easy, but the reality is very different. Every step of the way is paved with speed bumps, and progress is slow and uneven, with plenty of setbacks.*

When a celebrity reveals an eating disorder to the public, a patient may see it almost as an endorsement of her behavior. The same goes for the other stars who come out about their eating disorders. They inadvertently give the impression that having an eating disorder is trendy, something every cool kid should try. Of course, the large majority of kids, teens, and now adults who try to restrict their food to anorexic levels will quickly give up out of sheer hunger. There's that small minority, however, who are already leaning in that direction. They're the ones that end up being seduced by the glamour of a celebrity eating disorder. They try starving themselves and find they're good at it.

Actors and models appearing on talk shows make it sound as if getting over an eating disorder is quick and easy, but the reality is very different. Every step of the way is paved with speed bumps, and progress is slow and uneven, with plenty of setbacks.

To make progress, a patient has to make some difficult changes. I've had to do that in my life, too. I tell my patients, "You know what, when I had to make those changes it felt impossible. It took me a long time and I made a lot of mistakes." Sometimes my patients say I must be reading their minds, but I always tell them that my intuitive understanding of them comes from years of treating individuals with eating disorders. I also remind them that I still need to know what they're thinking for our therapy to work.

# Talking About It

There's a general tendency to walk around on eggshells when dealing with a family member who has an eating disorder. Other family members worry about saying the wrong thing or doing something that somehow triggers the eating disorder behavior; however, the more they treat the patient as a person and not an illness, the greater the chance of recovery. The more they tiptoe around the problem and are afraid to talk about it, the more the patient is getting reinforcement of the eating disorder behavior.

My patients know that what they say to me is completely confidential—they can tell me anything. When it comes to how they talk about their therapy with their family, I tell them that they don't have to treat our sessions as top secret. Being secretive about what goes on in therapy—refusing to say anything about it—can lead to the therapy taking on a life of its own, to the point that it becomes more the focus for the rest of the family than it needs to be. Still, it's important that patients feel comfortable with what they reveal, and don't try to use therapy as a way to live up to the expectations of others. When parents and loved ones ask, "How did it go?" I tell my patients to trust their own feelings and to reveal as much or as little as they want. If they want to keep things private, that's their right. I suggest giving generic, noncommittal answers such as "It was a good session" or "I really got a lot out of it," and not to feel that they have to provide anything further than what they're comfortable with.

---

*Tiptoeing around the problem will only reinforce the eating disorder identity and the behavior that supports it.*

---

# Responsibilities and Choices

It's important that family and community learn to stay out of the food, weight, and appearance issues. You know that the patient has anxiety issues. You know that the patient is a perfectionist. You know that the patient tends toward obsessive behavior. And you know that ritualized eating behavior is part of an eating disorder. You also need to know how important it is not to validate these tendencies and behaviors, that if you start getting too involved with the food the patient is eating—or not eating—you will reinforce the behaviors. You set up a situation where food can be used as a very powerful method of self-destruction. Let the individual be responsible for her food. Respect her choices—and ask her to respect your choices as well.

At the same time, it's important to avoid a situation where a child can use the parents by pretending that everything is okay, when clearly it's not. For example, if a child starts to raid the kitchen for the binge food and the parents not only keep quiet about it but go out and buy the food again, the behavior gets reinforced. I have even watched parents lock the refrigerator, hide food in the house, keep food in the trunk of the car—all to keep it away from someone who's either bulimic or a binge eater.

Similar situations arise with weight and appearance issues. Someone with an eating disorder might ask, "How do I look in this?" If you say good or bad, your comment is reinforcing the behavior either way. Staying neutral is more helpful. A good response in this situation is "I really don't want to get pulled into any questions about body image or appearance." This answer helps you stay out of the issue and helps the patient focus on her own internal values instead.

---

*Let the individual be responsible for her food. Respect her choices—and ask her to respect your choices as well.*

---

A lot of things that are said to people with eating disorders are incredibly harmful, even when they're said casually or when trying to help. The person with an eating disorder already has a negative self-image and a mind filled with negative words. All these statements simply reinforce the negativity and feed into the destructive eating disorder language.

### Food Statements

Why don't you just eat?

What's so hard about not overeating?

Do you really want to eat that?

Are you having more!!

When are you going to stop?

### Weight Statements

You look like you put on a few pounds.

What's your weight?

You weigh how much!?

### Appearance Statements

You look so much better.

You look just terrible.

You're all skin and bones.

I wish I could look like you.

You're disgusting.

### Other Harmful Statements

What did we do to deserve this?

How can you be so selfish?

We have paid so much money for treatment
    and you're still not better.

You are driving us crazy.

# The Outsiders

What if you found your best friend vomiting in the bathroom?

What if you found your wife weighing herself every day and looking like a skeleton?

What if you found your sister running miles each day and never eating anything?

What if you found your husband losing more than 15 percent of his body weight and he didn't have any illness?

What if you found your roommate in the middle of the night bingeing on the entire contents of the refrigerator?

What if your best friend has stopped talking to you and has closed you off from all avenues of communication?

What if your wife began having mood swings and extremely depressing thoughts that kept her in the bedroom all day?

What if your sister moved away, was later found dead, and you discovered from her therapist that she had been struggling with anorexia and exercise bulimia for ten years and you never knew?

What if your husband lost his job and was admitted into an eating disorder program for treatment?

What if your roommate stopped going to work, stopped paying rent, and refused to get out of bed?

What if you found that your best friend has an eating disorder and that's why she was constantly vomiting and had closed you out of her life?

What if you found that your wife's weight loss, mood swings, and depressing thoughts were caused by an eating disorder called anorexia nervosa?

What if you found yourself filled with guilt about your sister's death and your lack of awareness of her eating disorder?

What if you found yourself not being able to pay for treatment any longer and you've used up all your money to save your loved one's life?

What if you found that your roommate has a binge eating disorder and you can't do anything to change her behavior or convince her to seek treatment?

The problem is that there are often no clear-cut answers to any of these questions. The scenarios here are more about the best friend, the spouse, the sibling, or someone extremely close to the individual who has an eating disorder. These "outsiders" are the individuals who have difficulty in two ways: the struggle when they don't know what is going on and the struggle of what to do when they do know.

The outsiders are never handed a "how-to" book in detecting and dealing with someone with an eating disorder. The signs, symptoms, and behaviors are hard to discover. Far too often their loved one struggles for years before they are found out or disclose their illness.

Prior to knowing that their loved one has an eating disorder, the outsider may feel frustration, anger, or even resentment because they just do not understand what is going on. After the outsider finds out, they may feel guilt from the earlier expressed feelings. They struggle with wanting to change the situation and feeling helpless at the same time.

At this point communicating with their loved one and coping with the fact that they have an eating disorder becomes overwhelming. This is when the "outsiders" need to seek help. Seeking help means first finding out more about eating disorders and support programs. If the person with the eating disorder is not ready for treatment, you can literally stand on your head and there is nothing you can do about it. If that is the case, the outsider can always receive help, which will eventually allow an opening for other forms of treatment to occur.

Finally, when do you support? When do you intervene? And when do you let go? These are questions that have independent answers based on each individual's situation.

# Family Support Communities

I find families get the most benefit from a two-part approach: family sessions with a therapist and the patient, and if possible, participation in family support communities.

Family support groups are one approach. They can include anyone—parents, siblings, relatives, spouses, fiancés, friends. All that's needed is a willingness to listen. A typical support group will include people who are dealing with patients at every level. Most participants have a loved one who is in some sort of treatment for an eating disorder. The patient could be at any stage, from very sick to well into recovery. Sometimes the group has participants who are hoping to get someone into treatment; other participants are there reluctantly, not really willing to admit that a loved one has a serious problem. The mixture of people in a support group is really valuable, because it gives the group a variety of inputs and perspectives. Those who have been dealing with the issues longer can share their experiences—both positive and negative—with those new to the eating disorder world.

## Family Sessions

I try to take what the family members gain from their outside support communities (that includes online support, books, and informative videos for those who don't have direct access to a support group) and apply that to our family sessions. Within the family sessions they learn that the focus isn't really on patients, but on all the participants. I ask the family members

---

*Sharing stories of recovery and also of relapse in a support group helps everybody realize that eating disorders are complex and confusing, and that the path out isn't necessarily a straight line—it's curvy and filled with speed bumps.*

---

questions like "How are you taking care of yourself?" and "What are you doing to work on your own recovery?" What we find is that parents and others have to go through their own process of recovery while their child goes through theirs. Sometimes a child will never get into treatment or will never really recover. The parents and others still need to have their own recovery to learn to let go, move on, and continue to support their loved one in any way they can. Through acceptance and understanding, support empowers the family to look into their own issues separately and distinct from the patient's.

# The Language of Eating Disorders

Therapists and support communities can help families learn how to communicate and understand the language of eating disorders. They learn how to avoid the traps of no-win answers to the constant questions asked: "Do I look fat in this?" "Am I beautiful?" Until the patient learns to change her perspective, you can't give a good enough answer. If you say, "Yes, you're beautiful," the patient will accuse you of lying. If you say something like "You have beautiful eyes," she'll twist it to mean she has an ugly nose. Once they realize this, though, family members can learn to reply in ways that raise self-esteem but also focus on the inner self, not on external appearance. Focusing on positive characteristics, talents, aspirations, and so on draws attention away from body image and back to the person within.

What I find with my patients is that when the family members have their own outlet for support, that's a benefit for the patient as well. I recommend that families seek outside therapy, whether it be individual or couples therapy. This helps the families learn to understand themselves better and takes some pressure off the patients. Many patients have told me, "My parents are finally off my back." When family members have their own therapeutic outlets and finally have their own space to vent, patients can then feel as if they have their own therapy, which somehow levels the playing field.

To help the family and the community know that I'm an ally not just for the patient but for them as well, I use a familiar concept used in addiction therapy called the three Cs:

- You didn't *cause* it.
- You can't *control* it.
- You can't *cure* it.

The three Cs are a great way to help take the guilt and blame out of the eating disorder experience.

Family members didn't cause the problem. That might sound false, given that I've talked a lot about the role of family conflict in eating disorders. But not everyone who grows up with family conflict or divorced parents gets an eating disorder.

Family members also can't control the eating disorder. They may try to, by getting very involved with the patient's food. If the patient has anorexia, they may be constantly pushing food on her. If the patient has bulimia, they may provide the binge food. If the patient is obese, they may make comments like "You know what's going to happen if you eat that." Engaging with the language of eating disorders as a way to try to control the disorder doesn't help. Finally, family members can't cure the disorder—only the patient can do that.

# Conflict in Recovery

## Marital Conflict

When spouses or significant others become part of the patient's treatment, conflict often arises. There can be a lot of disagreement within the relationship about whether a problem truly exists and what to do about it. Spouses or significant others, just like parents, can have trouble understanding why the partner can't just be the person they married or began dating. A spouse or partner often takes on a parental role and treats the patient like a child or an invalid. In fact, the spouse will often say to the patient, "You're such a child," as well as other very parentlike things, such as "You're not eating enough," or "You're not doing what the doctor said," or "I expect you to behave yourself in front of my parents at the dinner table."

Statements like that can reinforce the illness for the patient because now the partner or spouse is attentive and caring. When improvements take place and the spouse begins to back away, wellness isn't reinforced and the patient begins to wonder, "Do I want this illness or don't I?"

I try to get the spouse or partner into the picture right from the start so I can get a clear idea of the relationship and so they can see who I am and what my approach is like. When therapy starts off including them, I find we make better progress and there is less conflict at home.

## Family Conflict

All too often I see families in conflict over whether a problem even exists. This occurs most often in a divorce or separation situation, where parents may be playing out their own conflicts and battling each other for control. Situations like that can put the therapist in a real hot seat, because one parent wants me to succeed and the other wants me to deny that there is a problem. After a while, you don't really know who you're treating anymore. Each parent tells you a different story, and you hear a third story from the patient.

What I've learned over the years is that, whenever possible, it's best to call in both parents and all immediate family members right from the start—no matter what the marital status. That initial meeting is extremely important, because it helps us to start out on the same page. I give them an idea of who I am and I get an idea of who they are. I ask each person to tell me what he or she sees as the problem. I'm very careful to just listen and not judge or take sides. Setting the stage at the first family session is imperative. My goal is to be objective and fair but also understanding.

In many cases, I won't be able to arrange a family meeting with both parents and the patient. Sometimes one parent is missing due to death or distance (both physical and emotional). In families where both parents are physically available, whether or not they're living together, I still often have trouble getting the father figure to come in. Part of this is that fathers, even today, expect mothers to handle the health issues of the children. Part of it is that the fathers of many of my patients just don't have a lot of time for their families. They're successful professionals who are very busy with their work and may also spend a lot of time traveling on business. A big part of the reluctance, though, isn't lack of time or love for their child. Fathers seem to be less interested in the process of treatment and much more interested in the bottom line: "When will my child get better?" By that they really mean "When will my child gain weight?" I explain that the weight gain they want to see so badly won't start to happen until later on in treatment. I also explain that there's no blame here—there's nobody who needs to be fired for causing the illness.

I always remain proactive and encourage fathers to participate as much as possible. If the father is uninvolved in the treatment, he may end up feeling left out. If the father can't or won't come to see me, I'll find some method of communication so he knows he's an important part of the treatment team.

If the father does participate, that's a very good sign. What's even better is when the whole family is involved—both parents, other kids, even grandparents and aunts and uncles. That tells me the whole family is united in really caring about the patient. It doesn't mean they all agree on what the problem is or what to do about it, but it does mean that they're willing to listen, get some information, and maybe learn how to communicate a little better.

Sometimes it's the patient who resists the idea of a family session. The patient may tell me her family doesn't want to participate. Sometimes the patient is actually scared to have the parents come in, because she's afraid of what they might reveal. If the patient hasn't been fully truthful with me, for example, she might be afraid her parents will tell me that she has been engaging in bulimic behavior much more often than she has admitted to me. As we establish more trust in the therapeutic relationship, that issue often fades away and the patient becomes much more willing to involve the family.

## Absent Families

Family conflict over the eating disorder can happen even when the patient doesn't want family sessions. A patient can be well aware that family members aren't really interested in participating, or that if they do come to a session, their own troubles will keep them from participating in a meaningful way.

This came out very clearly in the case of Tamara. Her parents had always been very distant, too caught up in their own constant fighting with each other. When Tamara began therapy for bulimia, her parents began to fight about her and less about each other. Each parent approached the problem from a different direction, and neither one agreed with her treatment program. They didn't want to acknowledge that there was an eating disorder at all. Instead, they both agreed that Tamara was the problem. They put all their internal issues, their anger, and their own inadequacies on her. Not surprisingly, Tamara internalized that blame and felt everything that was wrong not only in her own life but in her parents' failing marriage was all her fault. Tamara constantly heard all sorts of negative statements from her parents, things like "That therapist was a waste of time," "How could you spend so much money on treatment that isn't needed?" "How can you be so selfish?" and "What do you need treatment for?" Rather than becoming Tamara's allies in her treatment, her parents became estranged from her instead.

What Tamara's parents were doing, in a very destructive and thoughtless way, was venting their own problems and using Tamara as a target. The direct message from her parents, however, was that they were abandoning their support for her treatment.

When family conflict is really severe and the patient can't get away from it, the therapist has nowhere to go. When two parents are denying the problem, they create a lot of doubt for the patient to continue treatment. The parents will sabotage anything the therapist tries to do. Fortunately, Tamara is an intelligent and resilient person. When she got old enough to get away from day-to-day contact with her parents, she was able to make progress in therapy. Her recovery was long and marked by a lot of setbacks, but today Tamara is an independent woman.

When the family is absent, patients can be very much on their own. When someone who was once the patient's major caregiver is lost through estrangement, distance, death, or some other reason, the loss can trigger the return or start of an eating disorder, because the patient's whole sense of identity is shaken. For anyone, there's a tremendous emotional void left when the major caregiver is no longer there. Coping with the death of a parent, for instance, is difficult for all of us— nothing in our lives can really prepare us for it. For someone with an eating disorder, the illness can fill that emotional void with something familiar and comforting. Because the caregiver is no longer there to provide protection, safety can be found again by retreating back into the eating disorder.

The loss of a major caregiver can also trigger an eating disorder for the first time. This is often because food and nourishment are associated with caregiving. When the caregiver is no longer there, a vulnerable person may compensate for the missing care by eating in a disordered way. Without a caregiver to keep an eye on them or direct them onto a healthier path, the eating disorder can become their new identity.

A common trait among many individuals with eating disorders is that they are very good at taking care of everyone else but themselves. They often lack the skills of self-understanding and self-care, because they have ignored their own needs for so long. When a major caregiver is lost, these individuals often have to learn how to re-parent themselves and learn new self-care skills, because now there's nobody else who's going to do it for them. At this time in the treatment, the therapist has to help patients understand what they're going through and teach them how to nurture themselves, so they don't have to sabotage themselves by repeating their old scripts. I encourage patients to learn how to reach out to other people and talk about their feelings, rather than directing their feelings toward food.

If trust is established in the therapeutic relationship, patients talk

*Recovery is rarely quick and easy, even with a highly
supportive family and community of caring people; but
with the willingness of both the individual and the support
of community, it is possible.*

about their loss in the safety of that space, because they don't feel safe anywhere else. I know that feeling very well. When my father died, I didn't have any way to express how I felt. I just shut down instead. It was only several years later, when I visited a favorite place in Baja, California, where we both had often gone to fish, that I was finally able to accept that he wasn't there anymore. I opened that sad void, and out poured all the tears and emotions that I had been shutting out. I have recognized similar reactions in patients and friends when there has been the loss of a loved one.

Another situation can also arise—there's a family, but they won't or can't be involved. The family might be completely uninterested, or unable to acknowledge that a problem exists, or cut off from the patient, or absent due to death or abandonment. Some patients have been distanced from their families for so long, or had so little family to begin with, that they have been completely on their own for a long time. These patients are very independent individuals. The situation can be very difficult to treat, because the patient doesn't believe anyone can tell them a better way. They'll say to me, "Who are you to tell me to take care of myself better or change things? I've come this far doing it my way and I'm fine." Of course, these patients are not fine—if they were, we wouldn't be having the conversation. What they're really saying to me is that they've achieved some sort of very precarious balance and they're petrified about making any significant changes.

# TEN

# The Trauma Self

*Sometimes an individual* has had a major traumatic experience—or a series of them—that is so severe it takes away his or her original identity. The external traumas become the self. An eating disorder then becomes a desperate attempt to regain some sort of identity, damaged as it may be, and restore a fragile sense of control. Someone who develops an eating disorder as a result of serious trauma is actually showing a certain amount of psychological resilience by finding an identity at all.

The traumatic experience is generally defined as long-term, serious physical, sexual, or psychological abuse, or all of the above. Often the trauma is deeply hidden from the therapist—it can take months or even years of trust-building between the therapist and the patient before even a hint of the story comes out. When it does, some of the underlying causes of the eating disorder are revealed. This is progress, because there's no way someone can let go of an eating disorder identity without first recognizing and healing from the trauma.

*Trauma is often a root cause of an eating disorder.*

# Laurel's Story

When I first met Laurel, she had been suffering from anorexia for sixteen years. She had bounced from therapist to therapist, but nobody had been able to help her for long. Despite an extremely critical, fractured, and unhelpful family, and despite her illness, Laurel had managed to finish college and go on to graduate school, supporting herself all the way.

In my office, Laurel was almost mute—she couldn't find the words to tell me about herself and why she had come to see me. Rather than telling, Laurel showed. She had brought along some beautiful collages she had made, art that expressed her feelings in pictures better than she could in words at that time. Something about Laurel's art spoke to me, saying that here was someone in desperate need of help and willing, even if she couldn't say so, to do what it took to get well.

Laurel took a long time to find her voice. When she finally did, her story painfully emerged. It was a tragic one, involving physical, sexual, emotional, and verbal abuse, with a series of rapes, an unwanted pregnancy ending in a miscarriage, self-harming behavior, and much more—all against a backdrop of betrayal by trusted friends and a complete lack of support from her family. Laurel's original identity as an intelligent young woman with real artistic talent had been ripped from her; her self-identity had become the trauma self. She eventually discovered that she could substitute severe anorexia, along with bulimic behavior involving both vomiting and overexercising, for her displaced real identity.

Being labeled with an eating disorder led Laurel deeper into the illness—and deeper into increasing isolation and depression. She avoided relationships of any sort. Her long history of abuse by family members and strangers made her fearful of intimacy and physical contact, and her lack of trust made it hard for her to have friends or even acquaintances. Laurel was so ashamed of the abuse she had been through that she couldn't find a voice to describe it. She expressed her self-hatred outwardly by self-harming behavior, especially through cutting.

When Laurel started telling me her story, she realized that there were large gaps in her memory of her adolescent and young adult years. These were times when things were so bad that she had simply blanked them out. Some of her repressed memories began to come out very painfully as we worked together, which led to flashbacks and recurring bad dreams, along with some lapses and relapses, and a return of some self-harming behavior.

The path to recovery is often bumpy, of course, but Laurel's was bumpier than most. I wouldn't let Laurel slip away from me, however, and gradually she realized that she didn't have to remember and relive every trauma, and punish herself for them all over again, to heal. She learned gradually that she no longer had to feel guilt, shame, or a sense that she was to blame for all that had happened to her. These feelings and memories might never really go away, but they could be moved aside so that she could go forward with her life.

The same was true of her eating disorder. Once Laurel began to see that the eating disorder identity was her refuge from the trauma, but not her true identity, the intensity of the pain started to lessen. The gradual decrease of pain occurred over many months and was aided specifically by Laurel's passion for art. Rather than experiencing her pain concretely, her artwork allowed her to create abstract trauma images to explain her voiceless identity. When I first pointed out her artistic talent, Laurel was astonished. She saw her art as a projection of her trauma self, something that was unpleasant and negative to look at. She saw only darkness, never a light at the end of the tunnel. Her art continued to change in color, form, and texture. Through discussions about her changing images, the artwork itself became less complex and brighter. Her voice also sounded stronger and less fearful. She continued to deny her talent, but the art spoke for itself. The trauma self began to emerge more clearly in the drawings and the different layers of the colors used. Laurel began to admit openly that some of her art was actually quite deep and beautiful. This allowed a new voice to enter into her therapy. Her talent ultimately evolved into her new identity. Her true self was finally able to reemerge from the wreckage of trauma and the eating disorder.

Laurel's insights took a long time to happen; her recovery from her eating disorder wasn't quick or easy, and her life even today isn't always easy. Laurel's recovery happened despite a lack of community and even though the people who mattered most to her had given up on her. Her recovery was difficult, yet it happened. Her story reminds me every day that there is hope for everyone who suffers from an eating disorder.

# Trauma

Trauma comes in many forms and doesn't have to be related to abuse or horrifying experiences. Trauma can be the death of a loved one, moving away from home, or changing employment; sometimes it's the sense of being lost that comes from having no real identity.

As the layers of the disorder get peeled back in therapy, all sorts of hidden behavior and repressed experiences come out. When the patient gets that close to the core issues, there's often a return to eating disorder behavior—dropping or gaining weight—and sometimes a return to or the start of self-destructive behavior such as cutting or burning.

## Katherine's Story

Recently I thought I was doing really well with Katherine, a patient who struggles with compulsive overeating. She was losing weight, back in school, buying new clothes, and feeling more confident about herself. Suddenly she collapsed and returned to all sorts of binge overeating behaviors. She was close to hitting rock bottom and I started to get panicky.

---

*As the layers of the disorder get peeled back in therapy,*
*all sorts of hidden behavior and*
*repressed experiences come out.*

---

What had I missed? In my experience, a sudden lapse back into a severe eating disorder can indicate that we're getting close to a core trauma. That can be a very frightening prospect for a patient, and it can make her retreat back into the safest place she knows—her compulsive overeating. The eating disorder is a way to distract me from the core issues and toward just treating the symptoms.

I knew there had to be something serious that was triggering Katherine's behavior, but what? At this point she stopped talking in our sessions. She withdrew into herself, responded only with head nods, and watched the clock all through our time. At the end of our hour, she just stood up, said "Bye," and walked out. I don't do well with silent sessions. The silence upsets me, because I know that the silence only traps the patient further in a dark place, a space where she becomes voiceless.

The answer came when Katherine's mother mentioned an upcoming visit from distant grandparents. I asked Katherine if the visit might have anything to do with her collapse. Katherine finally spoke and told me she had been molested by her grandfather when she was five. That certainly explained the current collapse and also revealed the root cause of her eating disorder and current suicidal behaviors. Katherine had been living with a very deep and shameful secret for a very long time. She felt she could trust me enough to share this secret she had never told anyone before.

Telling me about the experience was a difficult step for Katherine. There's a sort of myth about therapy that says simply revealing all traumatic events at once to the therapist will make the patient magically heal from the trauma. Many therapists actively promote the myth after a patient has gotten something traumatic "out into the open." I help my patients set boundaries on how much to share at one time. Simply purging words that aren't connected to feelings leaves them feeling empty—and purging secrets with the feelings still attached and unprocessed can make them collapse into an abyss. When dealing with trauma, going slowly, and processing the emotions as we go along, is more effective.

I tell my patients very frankly that talking about bad things doesn't magically make the bad feelings and eating disorder symptoms go away.

Talking about traumatic events may very well make them feel worse and could trigger a return to disordered eating. They still need to discuss the traumas. I emphasize that the patient needs to feel surrounded by a sense of safety for this exploration to occur without harming her with post-traumatic memories.

Katherine's collapse didn't instantly stop once she revealed her history of sexual abuse. Over the next couple of weeks, however, her emotions stabilized and we started to move forward again. We still had to deal with the problem of her sexually abusing grandfather, who was about to arrive for a long visit. Because I had met several times with Katherine's mother and felt she would take the problem seriously, Katherine and I agreed to reveal the abuse to her. Her mother believed her at once. She had had unspoken suspicions all along and Katherine finally confirmed them. The visit from the grandparents was canceled.

# Trauma and Families

Not every family is supportive. Trauma such as sexual or physical abuse is bad enough, and it's made worse by shame and secrecy. When a patient reveals abuse, the therapist often feels the need to do something about it. Often, however, the family won't support the patient's version of events. Families have a very strong tendency to deny or minimize the big four of abuse—sexual, verbal, emotional, physical. What might seem genuinely minor to someone else, or what someone else would rather see as minor than deal with, can be extremely important to the patient. Family members often say the patient misinterpreted an innocent action, or they minimize the importance of what happened, or blame the victim, or deny anything happened at all. By refusing to acknowledge that something traumatic occurred, they're basically telling the patient she's nuts, or a liar, or both. That can become extremely disruptive and is not really helpful— it often makes the patient shut down completely and lose everything that has been accomplished up until then. For that reason, I am very careful about discussing traumatic events and possible abuse with a patient's family. It can cause a lot more problems than it solves if the family can't cope with the information.

# Eating Disorders and Self-Harm

Eating disorders and anxiety go hand in hand, because the eating disorder is a way to keep the anxiety under control. Sometimes that duo can turn into a threesome with the addition of another dangerous behavior—such as cutting or burning, also known as self-harm, self-injury, or self-inflicted violence. Cutting can be a form of external or self-induced trauma.

We can define cutting as the deliberate injury of one's own body in a way that causes tissue damage or leaves marks. Self-harming behavior can also include burning or branding with a hot object and other damaging actions, such as punching yourself or hitting yourself with an object (a hammer, for instance). I would also include some of the more extreme and self-mutilating forms of tattooing and multiple body piercings under the cutting category.

Often cutting behavior happens because individuals can't find a verbal way to express their feelings—they use their bodies instead. Self-injury and body hatred both tap into the underlying pain and express it in ways that words cannot. Even though self-harming behavior reveals serious trauma, it's not the same thing as suicidal behavior. The line can be thin, however, and people who cut themselves do sometimes go too far and cause serious damage or death. The therapeutic community has become much more aware of self-harming behavior in recent years, mostly because it has become very common.

---

*Cutting often occurs because individuals can't find a verbal way to express their feelings, so they use their bodies instead.*

---

The ways in which internal pain can be expressed externally through self-starvation and cutting are very clearly shown in Anna, one of my patients. Anna was twenty-three when she started treatment with me for anorexia and self-mutilation. She always wore baggy clothing and long-sleeved shirts, even in the warmest weather.

Anna told me that her eating disorder and cutting behavior had begun when she was thirteen. As we progressed with individual and family sessions, she revealed that she had been raped by a stranger when she was twelve. Through therapy, Anna came to realize that her self-starvation grew out of her desire to block out the memories and feelings created by that traumatic experience. Restricting her food intake and strictly controlling her body weight gave her something else to focus on obsessively. As another way to relieve the tension and anxiety caused by feelings and memories she couldn't block or control, Anna also engaged in self-injurious behaviors.

Anna's anorexia and self-harming behavior occurred while she was in what therapists call a dissociative state for cutters, where she felt detached from herself and her emotions. She felt disconnected from her body and from the sexual abuse. She visually displayed her internal pain by inflicting external wounds and starving herself to skeletal thinness.

I help patients deal with self-harming behavior in exactly the same way as I help with their eating disorder. We focus not on the behavior itself but on finding ways to cope with the underlying anxiety that is at the core. Just exploring the reasons for the self-harming behavior doesn't do much to reduce the behavior. Developing alternative coping mechanisms and learning to recognize anxiety and navigate through it are more effective.

Although it seems hard to believe, the pain from cutting is actually a way of lessening or calming intense emotional pain or anxiety. For some patients, it's a way of relieving feelings of emotional numbness—by cutting

*Many aspects of self-harming behavior have parallels to eating disorder behavior.*

yourself, you're finally feeling something. For others, however, cutting is actually a way of numbing themselves to emotional pain, and they may not even experience it as painful. For most, it's a way out when they feel too overwhelmed by their emotions to express themselves in any other way.

Other aspects of self-harming behavior also have parallels to eating disorder behavior. Cutting happens alone; it's a shameful secret that has to be hidden. People who cut themselves often cover the marks under long sleeves, long pants, scarves, even watches or bracelets, or they may harm themselves in places that can't be seen. As with eating disorders, the behavior causes guilt and shame. The behavior may get worse as time goes by, with more severe and frequent injuries.

Once Anna found ways through therapy to express the shame and guilt associated with her rape, her cutting and self-starvation eventually began to decrease. The process was long and slow, but today Anna is no longer engaging in self-harming behavior. She's learned to replace those old behaviors with more positive coping mechanisms, such as journaling. She now has a more positive relationship with herself.

## Drug, Alcohol, and Sexual Addictions

Alcohol and drug abuse are other forms of self-induced trauma. People with anorexia often see themselves as purists, controlling their weight through willpower alone. Even so, many misuse over-the-counter diet pills, diuretics, and laxatives as a way to restrict even more. They also rely heavily on caffeine, from coffee and other beverages and in pill form, and on other legal stimulants, herbal stimulants, and appetite suppressants. Some of my patients turn to cocaine, but most don't like the idea of using an illegal street drug.

My patients with anorexia rarely disclose their drug use to me at the start of treatment. That can be scary, because even over-the-counter drugs can be dangerous and even life-threatening. Once patients who use drugs start to eat again, they generally experience out-of-control hunger and bingeing episodes. At that point they're often very concerned about losing control, loosening up too much, and gaining too much weight.

---

*Regarding their bulimic behavior as out of control,
individuals with bulimia are far more likely to have
multiple addictions.*

---

Individuals with bulimia, on the other hand, already see their behavior as out of control—and they see themselves as out of control in other ways as well. These people are far more likely to have multiple addictions. What can make treating someone with bulimia very difficult is that she will often move from one addiction to another. While it's important to help someone with bulimia stop the binge/purge behavior, it's even more important to treat the underlying anxiety. If all a therapist does is treat symptoms, the patient will transition to a new set of symptoms once some progress starts to happen on the previous symptoms.

# Evan's Story

Evan came to me because at the age of forty-five he had suddenly become a compulsive binge overeater. He had gained a lot of weight in a short time, but what drove him to seek help wasn't the weight gain itself or that he had recently been fired from his job in the clothing industry. The rapid change in his behavior and weight had affected Evan's sexual function, and he was much more concerned about that. While he was still employed, Evan had begun an affair with a woman he met online. The affair didn't last. Although he was married, he began a string of other brief sexual relationships with women.

Evan quickly revealed to me that he had a past history of cocaine and alcohol abuse. The problems were severe enough that he had gone into a rehab program. The help he got there kept him drug- and alcohol-free for twelve years. Evan was proud that he still wasn't using drugs or alcohol. What he was doing instead, though, was using high-carbohydrate foods and sex as substitutes. He was still an addict, because the basic issues underlying his addictions—anxiety and obsessiveness—were still there.

Evan's first marriage had broken up over his drug and alcohol abuse. When he began therapy, he had been married to his second wife for eight years, and that marriage, too, was on the verge of collapse from his behavior. He and his wife were communicating only at the level of verbal abuse.

His earlier stay in rehab had helped Evan kick his earlier addictions, but they hadn't really gone away—they had simply gone underground. He had never developed positive coping mechanisms for handling anxiety and compulsiveness. His earlier solution had been to smother his anxiety with drugs and alcohol. He was doing the same thing now, with an eating disorder and sexual addiction.

To break out of this new cycle of self-destructive behavior, Evan needed to face his anxiety and learn new ways to channel his behavior into more positive paths. From the beginning of his therapy, Evan realized that his binge overeating was seriously affecting his health and ability to function sexually. That was a good starting point for exploring the underlying causes of the problem. Within a few months, Evan found another job. That was a big help in moving forward—instead of a lot of empty time that he filled with binge eating and sex, he now had a challenging new position and a chance for a fresh start. Evan still has a lot of work to do in discovering who he really is, and he may not be able to repair his marriage. He's feeling hopeful, however, and his episodes of bingeing and addictive sexual behavior are becoming much less frequent.

# Recovery and New Trauma

Trauma is often a root cause of an eating disorder. Even after an individual has recovered, a new trauma or major transition can trigger the disorder again. Pregnancy, for instance, can be very difficult for women who have recovered from an eating disorder. The crucial importance of good nutrition before and during pregnancy and while nursing brings their feelings about food to the forefront again for these women. At the same time, they're going through a very major transition, both physically and emotionally. For many people pregnancy is a time to celebrate and look forward with joyful anticipation. For people with eating disorders or those who have recovered from them, however, pregnancy can be a frightening time.

# Amber's Story

Amber was thirty-six and had struggled with bulimia for fifteen years. Her weight was so consistently low that she hadn't had a menstrual period for the last ten years; poor nutrition had left her with severely thinned bones (osteoporosis). She had also had irritable bowel syndrome and stomach ulcers that had caused serious bleeding more than once.

Amber had finally entered therapy after a hospitalization for her bleeding ulcers. She had revealed a past history of sexual abuse and was making slow progress when she fell in love with a very supportive man. Suddenly her therapy progressed much more quickly. In fact, Amber found a new identity in the commitment of marriage and stopped therapy.

Because Amber had been bulimic and hadn't had a period for so long, every fertility specialist she saw told her she would never be able to conceive. Miraculously, after three years of marriage her period spontaneously returned, and five months later Amber became pregnant. Her amazement and joy over the news soon gave way to major anxiety—in effect, pregnancy was a trauma for her. All sorts of fears came flooding back, along with frequent slips and lapses where she thought about returning to her bulimic behavior. Amber called me in a near panic to resume our therapy sessions.

Pregnancy had retriggered a lot of Amber's guilt and shame over her sexual abuse. And the physical changes of pregnancy also acted as triggers for Amber. The normal weight gain, increased appetite, and body-shape changes of pregnancy were associated, in her mind, with out-of-control eating and becoming fat. Her body image didn't include maternity clothes, a big belly, and swollen breasts. Her previous experience of sexual abuse left Amber sensitive about unwanted touching. She found it very hard to cope with the well-meant desire of other people—including her husband—to touch her pregnant belly.

As we talked, it also became clear that Amber feared the larger, permanent transition to being a mother, even more than the temporary changes of pregnancy. To help Amber deal with the pregnancy issues, we took a very rational approach. She read a book about nutrition during pregnancy, which helped her understand why she needed to eat properly and take in a lot more calories. It also helped her understand what to expect in terms of how her body would change and how much weight she would gain and how she would gradually return to normal after the birth. The bigger issue of transitioning into her new identity as a mother took a lot more discussion. Amber felt she had only just given up her eating disorder identity and adjusted to her new identity as a wife when she was very unexpectedly having to change identities yet again. She was well aware of her difficulties with transition and was concerned about her ability to take on the new parenting role.

Amber had learned a lot about herself during her earlier therapy. She had learned how to cope with ongoing anxiety, how to ignore the eating disorder voice, and how to handle her occasional slips and lapses. She was better prepared for the transition to motherhood than she realized—and for this transition she would also have the support of a loving husband. She continued to see me all through her pregnancy (which went very smoothly) and for a couple of years after the birth of her son. Despite all the transitions, pressures, and exhaustion of becoming a new mother, she never relapsed, and I feel confident going forward that she never will.

Any sort of trauma or important transition can be a trigger to someone who has recovered from an eating disorder, even when the illness is now long in the past. A desire to retreat back to the safe haven of the eating disorder when faced with something upsetting is a natural response. The difference is that people who are in recovery or recovered now have a better sense of their own identity and can handle the urge to return to the eating disorder. Will there still be slips and lapses, or possibly even a relapse? Yes, often to the point where the individual will feel the need to return to therapy. But fortunately, the progress made in earlier treatment usually means that the patient can quickly get past this new bump in the road.

*Serious trauma and abuse* can be major underlying causes for an eating disorder. They create terrible anxiety, guilt, and shame and destroy the individual's own sense of self. Recognizing the trauma and understanding how it relates to the illness can take a long time, and recovery for these individuals can be slow and full of obstacles. Even so, with patience and a willingness to heal, the trauma and the eating disorder can be overcome.

# EPILOGUE

# A Message of Hope

*. . . and the day came*
*when the risk it took to remain tight inside the bud*
*was more painful than the risk it took to blossom. . . .*

—ANAÏS NIN

*For more than half my life,* I have been treating individuals with eating disorders, learning from those who were brave enough to walk into my office and share their voices.

And I have learned.

I have learned that an eating disorder can affect anyone. Any age, any gender, any ethnicity, any religion.

I have learned that an eating disorder is less about control and more about identity.

I have learned that mutual trust and a willingness to change are key ingredients in the therapeutic relationship.

I have learned that being personal and interacting with my patients is key to guiding them toward a rational sense of self and, eventually, toward recovery.

Most of all, I have learned that I need to treat not just the eating disorder—that triad of food, weight, and appearance—but the individual as one, that other triad of body, mind, and soul.

Today we are faced with an eating disorder epidemic, an epidemic that takes in the full range of anorexia, bulimia, exercise bulimia, binge eating disorder, and compulsive overeating. The eating disorder spectrum spans two extremes: on one end anorexia, where individuals are emaciated and malnourished; and on the other end compulsive overeating, where individuals are morbidly obese. Our society sees extreme thinness as positive and something to strive for and extreme obesity as very negative and something to be avoided. The reality is far more complex, as the spectrum itself shows, because these extremes are about far more than just some standard or ideal; they are about identity.

We all want an identity that gives us a strong sense of self. But when that sense of self is vulnerable, we may be compelled to seek an identity based on the approval of others. When the search for self becomes defined by outside approval, that outer-directed identity can reach a tipping point that pushes it into something extreme, such as an eating disorder.

The eating disorder now has power over the individual. The disorder strips away any other identity from the person, finds a home within the voice, and moves right in. The search for a true identity ends, replaced by isolation, avoidance, and a confining solitude. The solitude becomes a way out: a safe space insulated from social pressures, life stressors, and whatever else seems too overwhelming and must be avoided. Within the solitude, the search for perfection continues. Individuals with eating disorders believe that perfection exists and is attainable. Wars have been fought for independence, yet people with eating disorders will battle long and hard to maintain their dependence on the illusion of perfection. In reality, what one is doing is declaring war on oneself, and lives are lost.

When *Dying to Be Thin* appeared on the shelves in 1987, I was hoping to raise awareness of the epidemic of eating disorders. Twenty years later, the epidemic is worse than ever, touching and ending more and more lives. I now want to use my voice to bring a new awareness to eating disorders, just as I ask my patients and their communities to use theirs.

If we can't really change the world, if we can't get rid of the media images of sub-zero supermodels and prejudice against obesity, what can make a difference in the eating disorder epidemic? Knowing that no one is truly alone in their struggle is the first step. Effective treatment and support are available, and recovery is possible. The struggle isn't the patient against the disorder, but rather the struggle to believe that there is a way out of this hell.

I define recovery, or the process of recovery from an eating disorder, as "regaining your self." Even with that hope, however, there is still a continuous struggle within ourselves, our loved ones, and our patients to take the risk to seek a new identity. I encourage all of you to take that risk, to regain your self.

# RESOURCES

Many of the dedicated organizations for people with eating disorders offer information and referral services. The list below contains organizations found to be objective and reliable.

Academy for Eating Disorders
60 Revere Drive, Suite 500
Northbrook, IL 60062-1577
847-498-4274
www.aedweb.org

The Alliance for Eating Disorders
Awareness
P.O. Box 13155
North Palm Beach, FL 33408
1-866-662-1235
www.eatingdisorderinfo.org

The Butterfly Foundation
www.thebutterflyfoundation.org.au

A Chance to Heal
1457 Noble Road
Rydal, PA 19046
215-885-2420
www.achancetoheal.org

Eating Disorder Information.com
www.eating-disorder-information.com

Eating Disorder Referral and
Information Center

23 Sandy Pointe, Suite 6
Del Mar, CA 92014
858-792-7463
www.edreferral.com

Eating Disorders Coalition
611 Pennsylvania Avenue SE #423
Washington, DC 20003-4303
202-543-9570
www.eatingdisorderscoalition.org

Eating Disorders Information
Network (EDIN)
2964 Peachtree Road NW, Suite 324
Atlanta, GA 30305
404-816-3346
www.edin-ga.org

Eating Disorders Online.com
www.eatingdisordersonline.com

The Gail R. Schoenbach F.R.E.E.D.
Foundation
(For Recovery and the Elimination of
Eating Disorders)
www.freedfoundation.org

Gurze Books
5145 B Avenida Encinas
Carlsbad, CA 92008
1-800-756-7533
www.bulimia.com

Healthy Place
www.healthyplace.com

International Association of Eating
Disorders Professionals (IAEDP)
P.O. Box 1295
Pekin, IL 61555-1295
1-800-800-8126
www.iaedp.com

My Self Help
184 Otis Street
Northborough, MA 01532
www.myselfhelp.com

National Association of Anorexia
Nervosa and Associated Disorders
(ANAD)
P.O. Box 7
Highland Park, IL 60035
www.anad.org

National Eating Disorder Information
Centre
ES 7-421
200 Elizabeth Street
Toronto, Ontario M5G 2C4
Canada
1-866-NEDIC-20
www.nedic.ca

National Eating Disorders Association
(NEDA)
603 Stewart Street, Suite 803
Seattle, WA 98101
206-382-3587
www.nationaleatingdisorders.org

National Eating Disorders Screening
Program
Screening for Mental Health, Inc.
One Washington Street, Suite 304
Wellesley Hills, MA 02481
781-239-0071
www.nmisp.org/events/nedsp/index.aspx

Ophelia's Place
P.O. Box 621
Liverpool, NY 13088
315-451-5544
www.opheliasplace.org

Pale Reflections
www.pale-reflections.com

Something Fishy
www.something-fishy.org

# "The Journey"
## Created by Laura D. McDonald, M.S.

*This workbook offers* the opportunity to enhance your recovery process from an eating disorder. The exercises and questions throughout can be used independently; however, it is highly recommended that this workbook be used as a therapeutic tool within the context of treatment. The designed activities will provide you with a new perspective on your eating disorder identity and your process toward recovery. To use this workbook effectively, please note that each section of questions and guided exercises corresponds with each chapter of the book and to the discussions within the chapters.

Living within the struggle of the eating disorder and trying to attain the process called "recovery" are both scary concepts to grasp. Your willingness to change is a powerful motivation to begin this workbook section, which is why it was written with the intention to aid and support you through the struggle and at the same time bring awareness to the process of recovery.

Prior to beginning the questions and exercises the required materials are:

- Journal or Notebook
- Pens, pencils, color pencils, pastels, or writing materials of your choice
- Drawing paper in various sizes

While you are completing each of the activities, give yourself permission to work at your own pace. Please allow time with guided support to process your answers, which have great significance on your road to recovery. Throughout the process of this workbook, keep in mind:

*"The journey of a thousand miles begins with one step."*

—Lao Tzu

# SECTION ONE: IDENTIFYING THE DISORDER

**Purpose:** To recognize your specific history, signs, and changes that are contributors to your eating disorder.

What has been the turning point/moment of clarity in your life that has created a desire for change?

When do you believe your eating disorder started and were there any significant events during that period of time?

In your own words how would you describe your eating disorder?

What have been the benefits and disadvantages of having an eating disorder?

How do you use your eating disorder as a mechanism to voice your feelings and emotions?

If you were to create a sign, what would it look like and what would it say? (Example): A sign in the shape of a stop sign that says in black letters "stay out!"

Complete the following statements:

*I look like . . .*

*I want to look like . . .*

*I need to look like . . .*

What have been appearance or behavior changes that you or others have noticed since the eating disorder began?

What is your current mood?

When you think of the idea of change, like recovering from an eating disorder, what specific fears or anxieties come to mind?

Rate your current level of motivation for recovery (on a scale of 1 to 10, with 1 being not at all ready and 10 being the most eager to get better).

In the past or currently have levels of your motivation to recover been prompted by outside influences (family, friends, treatment professionals) or a personal choice?

If you are motivated, what are the goals you want to concentrate on attaining?

# SECTION TWO: A DIVERSE DISORDER

**Purpose:** To gain a perspective of how cultural influences have contributed to your view of yourself.

Have the social pressures or cultural shifts of society, such as media (movies, television, magazines), the fashion industry, and/or marketing and advertising personally affected your distorted body image?

How has your age, gender, ethnicity, religion, and culture affected your eating disorder and your desire for wellness?

# SECTION THREE: ILLUSIONS OF PERFECTION

**Purpose:** To identify the parts of the *Obsessive Identity*. (Refer to Chapter Three—"These independent components—perfectionism, anxiety, and OCD—work together to produce the obsessive identity, which is a core component of the eating disorder identity")

How does anxiety affect your everyday life?

What triggers your anxiety?

How do you cope with your anxiety?

Do you believe that perfectionism does exist?

What role has perfectionism played in your life?

In chapter three, we discussed procrastination as a self-defeating behavior. How do you use self-defeating behaviors?

Does procrastination affect you? If so, how?

Does the theme of excessive activity (the opposite of procrastination) affect you? If so, how?

How does all-or-nothing thinking affect your thoughts?

What part or parts of the *Obsessive Identity*—Perfectionism, Internal and External Anxiety, or OCD—do you relate to and why?

# SECTION FOUR: SEEKING IDENTITY

**Purpose:** To approach the uncertainty of your identity.

What ten words would you use to define your own identity?

What are your strengths and weaknesses?

On a separate sheet of paper, draw a symbol that represents your identity, and write a word that describes your identity.

What identity do you exhibit to the outside world and what identity do you show to yourself?

What do you believe is your true identity?

Have you felt like a fraud in your life? If so, how?

How have your beliefs about a false identity misled you?

How does the phrase "not good enough" make you feel?

How have you strived for validation?

How does your eating disorder bring you comfort?

On a separate sheet of paper, draw an image of what your eating disorder looks like.

What are harmful statements outsiders have said to you regarding your identity?

What would you like to say to outsiders that you either cannot say or have difficulty saying?

How have you used control to sustain or defeat your eating disorder?

What part does trust play in giving up the concept of control?

How has your desire for control been an illusion?

# SECTION FIVE : BREAKING FREE

**Purpose:** To understand the transition from an eating disorder to recovery and how your identity evolves through change.

With words or images, describe the struggle with your eating disorder?

Imagine you had a mirror that could reflect back an image of your past self, present self, and future self. With words, describe what those three images would project.

With words or images, describe what freedom from your eating disorder looks like?

What expectations do you place on yourself?

What expectations do you place on others?

What does wellness mean to you?

What is your definition of recovery?

On a separate sheet of paper, draw a box that you have placed the gift of recovery in. What would the doors and windows of this box look like for you to access the contents?

If you were to write a letter to your eating disorder identity, what would it say?

If your eating disorder wrote back, what would be the response?

# SECTION SIX : PIRT–A NEW APPROACH

**Purpose:** To explore a new approach to the treatment of eating disorders.

What important components of Personal Interactive Rational Therapy (PIRT) would you like to apply to your own treatment in a therapeutic setting?

If you are not presently in treatment, what aspects of PIRT would you look for in a therapist or treatment team?

What parts of PIRT have been similar to past or present therapy?

What parts of PIRT have been different to past or present therapy?

# SECTION SEVEN: THE PROCESS
# OF RECOVERING THE SELF

**Purpose:** To clarify your road to recovery and process the negative and positive things that occur.

Where are you on your journey of recovery? Are you at the beginning, middle, or end of the process?

What words would you use to describe your recovery process?

On a separate sheet of paper, draw a map into and out of your eating disorder. What does the map look like?

What have been the obstacles on the road to recovery?

List your own personal

*Slips:*

*Lapses:*

*Relapses:*

*Collapses:*

How have you handled set-backs and what lessons have you learned from them?

How would you describe your triggers?

Describe both positive and negative transitions that have been, or continue to be, triggers in your life.

On separate sheets of paper, create a pros and cons list for "life without an eating disorder" and "life with an eating disorder."

## SECTION EIGHT: THE PASSION PURSUIT

**Purpose:** To create a purpose through passionate interests in order to fill the void of the eating disorder identity.

On a separate sheet of paper, draw an image of what "letting go of an eating disorder" means to you.

How would you define a passion?

What rocks your world?

What do you do with your open time?

What interests turn you off?

Create an "interests list" or an "anti-boredom" list.

What kind of things can you visualize that would decrease your focus on the eating disorder?

What would you like to add to your life that is presently not there?

If you could add one thing to your life what would it be?

What is blocking your pursuit for creating a passion?

What are some of your past talents, interests, or activities?

What would help you form a creative process to explore new interests and activities?

Once you find an established passion, what alternative passions would you also consider if you become bored or if you have too much open time?

How would you use your passion as a coping mechanism?

How would a passion create structure in your life if the eating disorder was no longer present?

# SECTION NINE: FAMILY & COMMUNITY IDENTITY

**Purpose:** To discover how the role of your external world affects your internal world.

What does your support structure look like?

My support system at this time is . . .

Describe your ideal support system.

Describe what a safe environment would be.

How would you define community?

Complete the following statements regarding relationships:

*I have a close relationship with . . .*

*I have a distant relationship with . . .*

*I am too dependent on my relationship with . . .*

*I am frustrated by my relationship with . . .*

*I want to build better communication with . . .*

*I want to establish a healthier independence with . . .*

Complete the following statements:

*Family is . . .*

*Home is . . .*

*Marriage is . . .*

*Divorce is . . .*

*Diagnosis is . . .*

*Death and loss are . . .*

*Parenting is . . .*

*Friendship is . . .*

*Abandonment is . . .*

*Betrayal is . . .*

*Rejection is . . .*

*Isolation is . . .*

*Guilt is . . .*

*Shame is . . .*

*Blame is . . .*

*Forgive is . . .*

*Comfort is . . .*

*Hope is . . .*

*Love is . . .*

*Purpose is . . .*

From the previous list of words, what has made the biggest impact on your life?

On a separate sheet of paper, create a collage of your family and friends using pictures to illustrate your community identity.

# SECTION TEN: THE TRAUMA SELF

**Purpose:** To look at the significance of painful moments in your life.

What was the best day of your life and what was the worse day of your life?

How would you define a trauma?

What have been your traumatic experiences?

How have transitions in your life been traumatic; for example, transitioning from an eating disorder identity?

How have you found support or closure in dealing with your trauma?

# SECTION ELEVEN: MESSAGE OF HOPE

**Purpose:** To allow yourself the opportunity to write your story
therapeutically.

On a separate sheet of paper or in your journal, write in your own words
a story titled "Regaining Your Self."

# INDEX